MW01596340

a guide to natural home remedies

a guide to **natural home remedies**

Liz Bestic

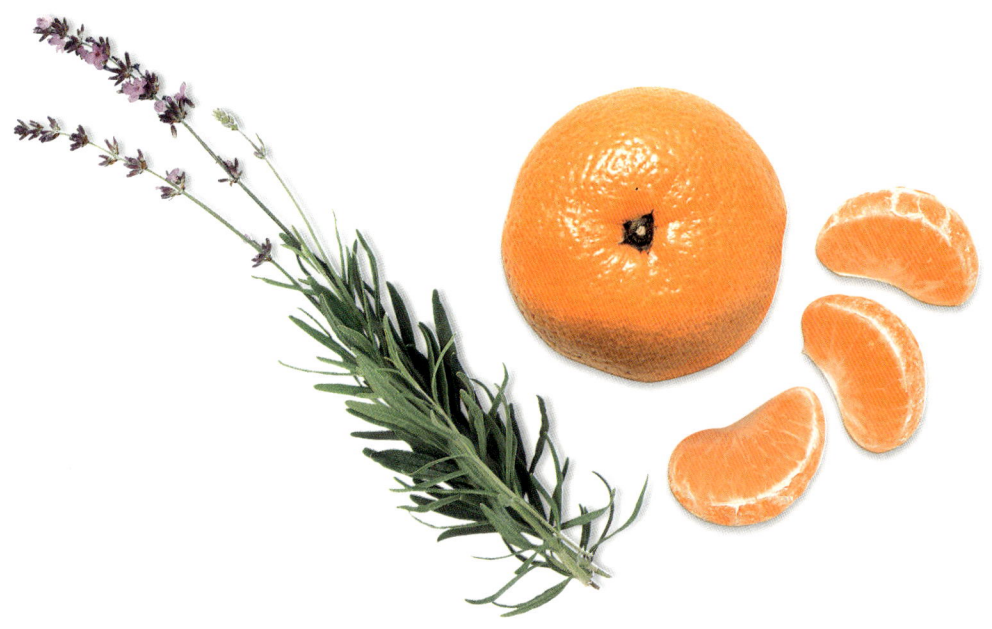

p

This is a Parragon Publishing Book
First published in 2002

Parragon Publishing
Queen Street House
4 Queen Street
Bath BA1 1HE, UK

Copyright © Parragon 2002

All rights reserved. No part of this publication may be reproduced,
stored in a retrieval system or transmitted, in any form or by any means,
electronic, mechanical, photocopying, recording or otherwise, without
the prior permission of the copyright holder.

ISBN: 0–75257–785–9

Printed in China

Produced by the Bridgewater Book Company Ltd

NOTE

Information given in this book is not intended as a substitute for medical
advice. Any person with a condition requiring medical attention should
consult a qualified practitioner or therapist.

ACKNOWLEDGMENTS

The publishers wish to thank the following for the use of pictures:
AKG London: 8, 9b; *A–Z Botanical Collection Ltd*: 45t; *Bridgeman Art Library*:
58b; *Corbis UK Ltd*: 13t, 22t; *Garden Picture Library*: 6b, 38b; *Getty Images*:
11t, 29t, 58t; *Hulton Getty*: 53; *Imperial War Museum, London*: 9t.

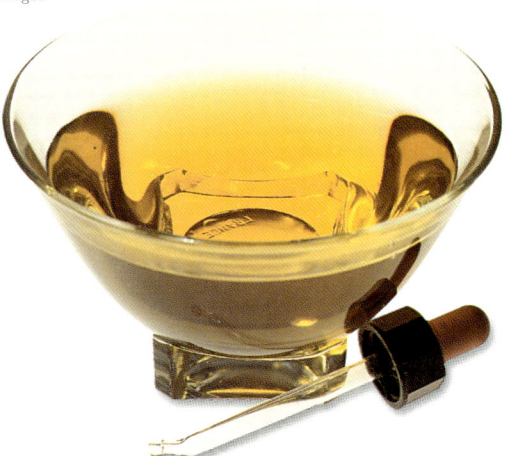

contents

Introduction

In the old days, when you had a sore throat your first reaction was probably not to call out the doctor but to head for the kitchen cabinet. There you would find the honey jar, spoon a liberal portion into some boiling water, add the juice and rind of two or three lemons and sip the warming concoction slowly. Honey and lemon is one of the best known and best loved home remedies and is still used today as a basis for many of the most famous over-the-counter medicines and throat sweets.

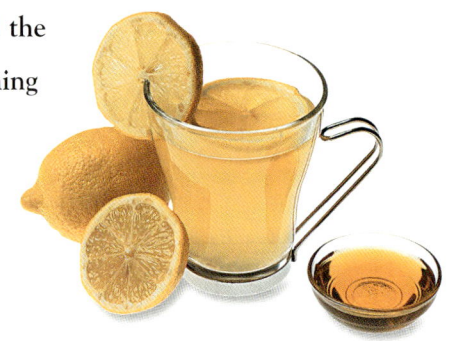

Nowadays, however, new technology and increasingly sophisticated medical advances have all but banished the old-fashioned home remedy to the archives of history. Most are dismissed as "old wives' tales" and yet many of these ancient remedies have been the subject of rigorous clinical trials. The humble garlic, for example, has probably been the subject of more scientific studies than any

A cupful of honey, lemon, and hot water will help to ease the symptoms of a cold such as sore throat.

other herb. We now know it is excellent for thinning blood, lowering cholesterol levels, and even curing the common cold. It is marketed as the new cure-all for a myriad of complaints.

Modern drugs can be life savers but they often have too many side effects to warrant their use for every little sniffle or stomach upset. Home and herbal remedies tend to heal without suppressing symptoms, and used in the correct dosage are perfectly safe and have no side effects. Herbs are easy to find and can be used in cooking or in salads. Some, which you can grow in your garden, can be ground up and used as inhalants or to perfume a bath. Others—which are more likely to be in your

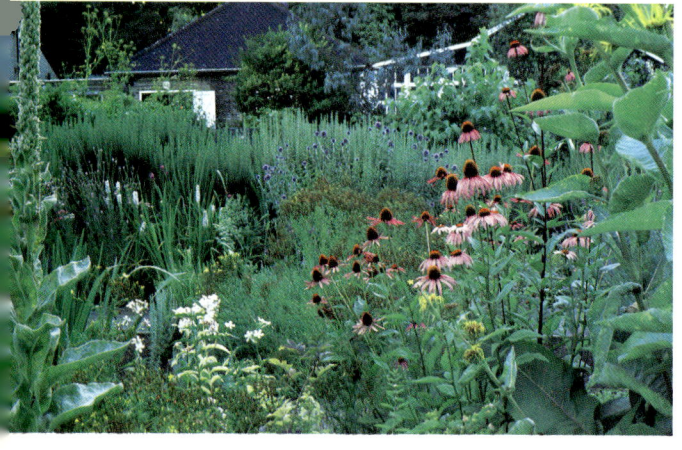

The modern herb garden can provide many home remedy possibilities. Herbs can be added to food or used as a treatment.

kitchen—can be added to cooking or made up into poultices and muscle rubs.

As the methods of testing the compounds contained in many natural remedies become more sophisticated, many cynics are beginning to sit up and take notice. And as more and more of our so-called "wonderdrugs" prove only to suppress symptoms rather than get to the root cause, it is little wonder that more and more people are now looking for a healthier option for everyday complaints. The beauty of home remedies is that they are accessible and easy to prepare. Many of the remedies contained in this book have been passed down through the generations by word of mouth—others have surpassed all expectations in clinical trials. Some you will remember from the old nursery rhymes. Remember when Jack fell down and broke his crown and Jill fixed it with vinegar and brown paper? It may have sounded a strange remedy for a bad head, but in fact this used to be a remedy for headaches and migraine!

Garlic has been the subject of many scientific studies.

How to Make Home Remedies

Compress

A compress is simply a piece of cloth soaked in a bowl of hot or cold herbal extract. It eases the strain of painful joints and muscles and can help to soothe skin rashes. Almost any herbs can be applied as a compress if you need to treat a problem locally. All you need to do is soak a piece of cheesecloth or lint in the herbal infusion of your choice and apply it to the affected area, renewing it as and when necessary.

Steam Inhalation

For steam inhalations, which are best for stressed or inflamed lungs, make up an infusion of the herb you want to use (essential oils can also be used) and add it to a basinful of hot water. Drape a towel around your head and the basin so that you keep the steam in, and inhale slowly and deeply for a few minutes.

Tincture

To make a tincture, put $4\frac{1}{2}$ cups of fresh herbs or $1\frac{3}{4}$ cups of dried herbs in a jar and add $2\frac{1}{4}$ cups of vodka (it acts as a preservative). Add a scant cup of water, seal the jar and store in a cool place for 2–3 weeks, checking and shaking it occasionally. Strain the liquid through a cheesecloth bag into a pitcher and then into sterilized bottles.

Infusion

To make an infusion to drink hot or cold, warm a teapot and add about $\frac{1}{4}$ cup of dried herbs or $\frac{1}{2}$ cup of fresh herbs. Pour $2\frac{1}{4}$ cups of hot water on the herbs. Cover the pot until the herbs have infused (about 10 minutes). Strain the infusion through a plastic tea strainer. Add a little honey or unrefined sugar. Drink a cupful. You can keep the remainder in a pitcher and store in the refrigerator for up to 48 hours.

History of Home Remedies

Home remedies have been around for thousands of years. Even these days about 30% of prescription drugs are still synthesized from plants. In fact, the word "drug" comes from an old Dutch word, *drogge*, which means "to dry"—which is how many plant medications were prepared.

Honey is one of the oldest remedies known—in the days of the ancient Egyptians it was used as a remedy for high blood pressure. Honey contains a huge range of vitamins, enzymes, proteins, and amino acids; it can actually be classified as a complete food. Honey not only lowers blood pressure but is also a key factor in transmitting nerve impulses.

Vinegar is another ancient remedy which has stood the test of time. Cider vinegar was used for treating ailments long before the expression "an apple a day keeps the doctor away" was coined. Apples contain pectin— a soluble fiber—as well as all sorts of vitamins and minerals. Cider vinegar is rich in potassium, which promotes cell growth, and for many years vinegar was believed to be the "fountain of youth." It can help high blood pressure and is excellent for curing cramp. Vinegar was also used by the ancient Assyrians to cure earache, and during the American Revolutionary and Civil Wars it was used as both an antiseptic and disinfectant.

The Chinese were big on home remedies and were one of the first civilizations to recognize ginger for its therapeutic properties. It was and still is used to combat nausea, boost the immune system and reduce inflammation.

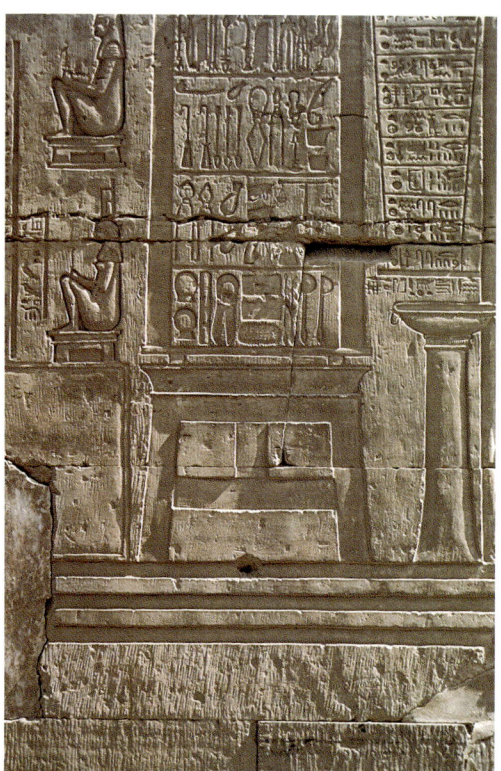

The ancient Egyptians used honey for high blood pressure centuries before the full range of its benefits had been scientifically analyzed. It contains a raft of vitamins and may be classified as a complete food. No wonder it is so useful in the battle against colds.

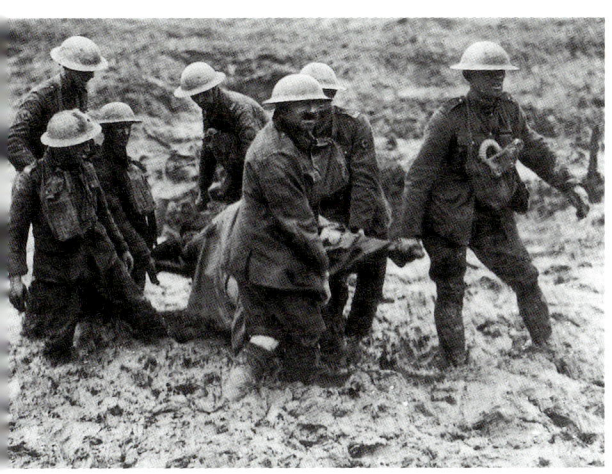

Some of the best home remedies were discovered on the battlefield. Garlic was used to dress wounds in the First World War.

For more than 2,000 years celery stalk was a remedy used by Chinese healers to treat high blood pressure. Recent research has shown that celery stalk does contain compounds that reduce high blood pressure by relaxing the smooth muscle lining the blood vessels.

Some of the best home remedies were discovered on the battlefield. During the First World War, for example, garlic was pounded in water and applied to wounds on a bed of moss as an accepted field dressing, while during the eighteenth century sailors used to thrust a piece of shag tobacco into a wound to staunch the bleeding!

So you can see that home remedies are an excellent form of first-line treatment. And although this book is not in any way intended to replace the advice of your doctor, by being more aware of the benefits of home remedies

Vinegar has many uses as a natural home remedy. It is rich in potassium and can help with cramp and high blood pressure.

you can begin to understand how to heal yourself.

Naturally, if symptoms persist, or you are in any doubt whatsoever about a health problem, you should always consult a professional. But before you pick up the telephone, you should use this book as a reference point for everything from smelly feet to the common cold. You will be surprised at what may be lurking in your kitchen cabinet that might just do the trick!

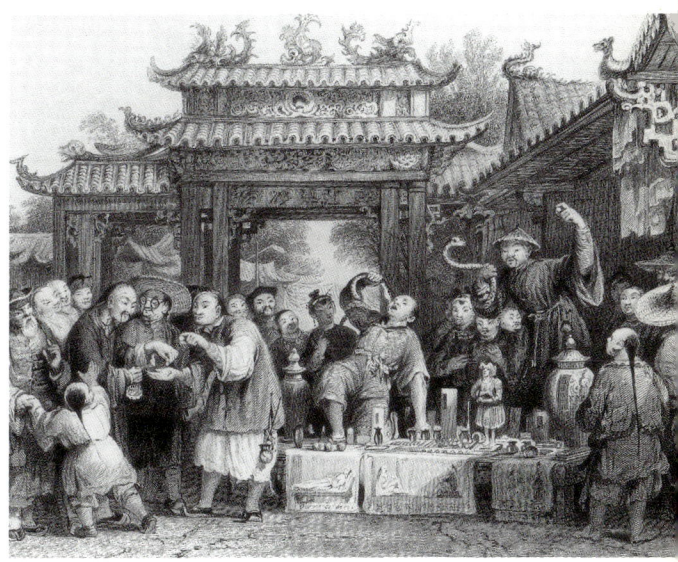

China has a long history of natural home remedy use, including celery stalk to reduce high blood pressure.

Burns, Scalds, and Sunburn

Although second- and third-degree burns require hospital treatment, mild first-degree burns are often superficial and can be treated at home. Any burn needs cooling down, so run tepid water directly onto the wound for at least five minutes to reduce the heat and give pain relief. For a chemical burn it is vital to keep flushing the skin with cold running water until well after the pain has subsided. Clean the burn of any grit or dirt very carefully, avoiding breaking the skin or blistered areas.

Remedies for Burns

Plain yogurt applied to a burn will keep it cool, or you can make up a soothing poultice from honey and yogurt. Adding crushed elderberries to the poultice will make it more effective or mash the leaves of the elder with a little butter and use it as a mild cream for the affected area.

Cucumber mashed to a pulp and mixed with glycerine makes a particularly wonderful moisturizing balm.

Cool the whole area with a cider vinegar splash and make sure the person who has been burned has plenty of fluids.

Try making a tea made from lemon balm, which will both calm the patient and provide further pain relief.

Flush the skin with cold running water for a while after a chemical burn—even after the pain has subsided.

Olive oil can bring effective relief to a painful scald.

Remedies for Scalds

Olive oil can bring immediate relief to a painful scald and will improve the chances of healing without blisters or scars. If you have any lavender or peppermint essential oils to hand, add these to the olive oil to help ease the stinging sensation around the wound.

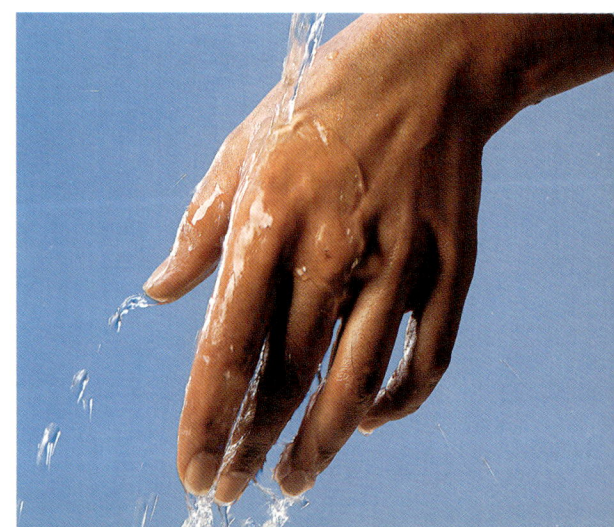

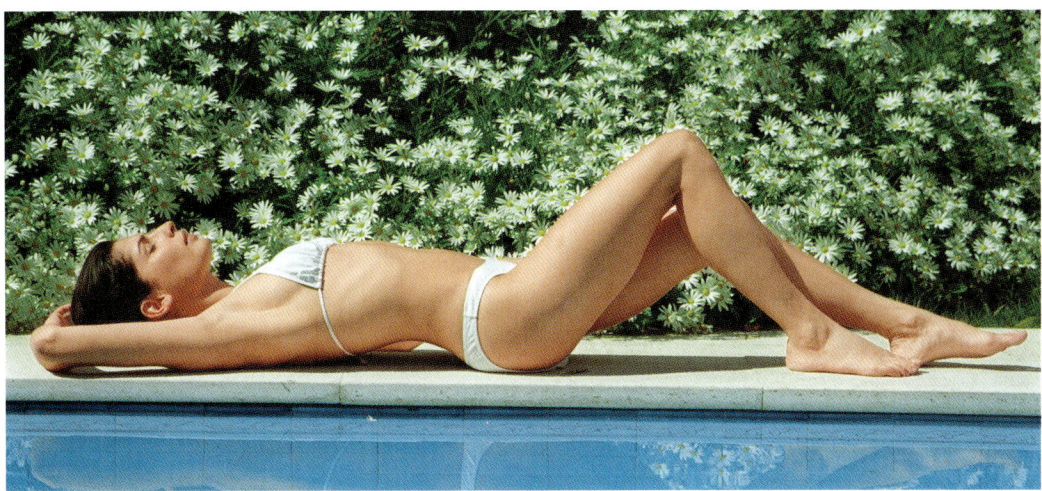

When sunburn spoils a holiday, natural home remedies made from lemon, cold tea, and baking soda can come to the rescue.

Remedies for Sunburn

For instant relief from sunburn, dab on a little lemon juice or soak a flannel in cold tea and place it over the affected area. For the kind of all-over sunburn that keeps you awake at night, try adding two tablespoons of baking soda to a cool bath and immerse your whole body in the water. You can also mash the pulp of a ripe avocado and smooth over the sunburnt area for a soothing effect.

Bathe your face in buttermilk or grate up some potatoes and apply to the sunburned area. The starch will cool and soothe the burn. Use cold peppermint tea as a mild wash to ease the stinging. Or you can try dissolving Epsom salts or baking soda in cold water and draping a cloth soaked in the solution over the affected area.

Milk of magnesia has been successfully used to treat sunburn, and mud or clay can ease the stinging pain.

Remedy for Chapped Skin

Fill a cheesecloth bag full of oats, then tie it up at the top and drop it in a cool bath, or soak it in warm water, squeeze it out and rub it over the chapped area during the day to ease the pain.

A cheesecloth bag filled with oats and soaked in a cool bath can be rubbed over areas of chapped skin to help relieve the pain.

FIRST AID
Bites and Stings

There is nothing more painful and irritating than being stung by an angry wasp or bitten alive by mosquitoes. It is vital that you have identified what has bitten you before using a home remedy, and if you are traveling abroad and are stung by an unknown flying creature it is always safest to seek medical advice. However, for the everyday type of insect bite or sting, ice-cold water or witch hazel are good first-line remedies.

Remedies for Bee Stings

Remove bee stings with tweezers (grasp the sting below the poison sac). Apply a paste of baking soda and cold water. A mixture of parsley juice and honey will also help to ease the irritation—crush the parsley leaves and stems to release the juice.

A cold, wet tea bag makes a marvelous poultice for bites and stings. Tea contains tannic acid, which helps to reduce swelling.

It helps to identify what you have been bitten by before using a home remedy.

Remedies for Wasp Stings

Cider vinegar or lemon will help to stop the irritation and itching. In the rare event of swallowing a wasp, drink a glass of cold water mixed with a teaspoon of salt. If you have been stung in the mouth, suck on ice cubes until the pain subsides. Mix cider vinegar with baking soda to make a poultice and apply directly to a bite. A cold, wet teabag makes a marvelous poultice—the tannic acid helps to reduce swelling. A paste of ground cloves and cold water can also help.

Remedies for Mosquito Bites

Rub neat garlic directly onto mosquito bites to prevent infection—and mosquitoes loathe the smell of garlic, so eat the rest of the clove raw! Honey and baking soda mixed together

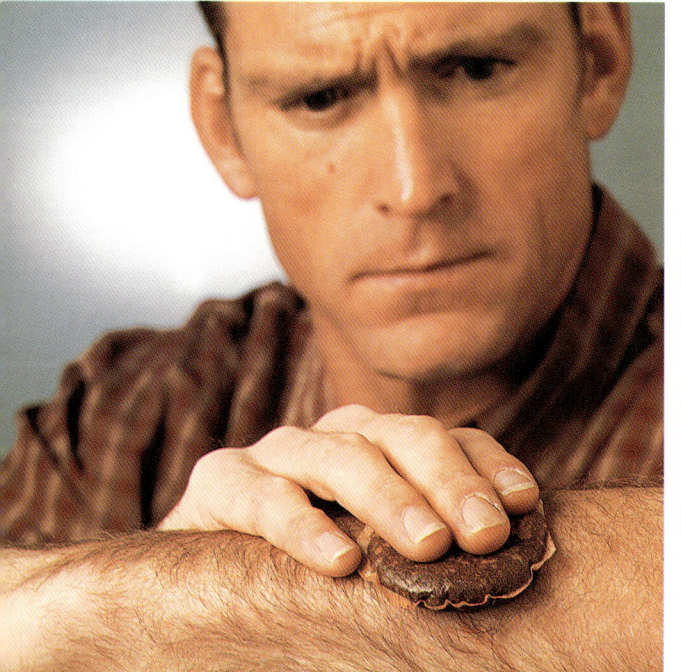

The pain of a jellyfish sting can be reduced by pouring seawater over the affected area for at least ten minutes.

can help the itchiness around the bite, or rub the rind of a lemon neat onto the site of the bite. Sprinkle dried lavender along your window sill to stop further attacks—the smell of lavender also instantly repels mosquitoes!

To make another mosquito repellent, tie together some dried lavender, peppermint, and catnip and secure it with a piece of thin wire. Light the bundle and keep it in a jar nearby. The smoke will mask your own smell and literally put the bugs off the scent!

If you are covered in bites, you need to break down the toxins which have been released into your body. Try drinking herb teas made from dandelion root, red clover or burdock.

Make a tincture of horseradish using half a cup of grated horseradish root and $2\frac{1}{2}$ cups of rubbing alcohol. Steep the root in the alcohol for 2–3 days. Shake the mixture up twice every day. Strain off the grated root and bottle the liquid. You can use the tincture for most bites and stings, minor skin wounds and any superficial infections.

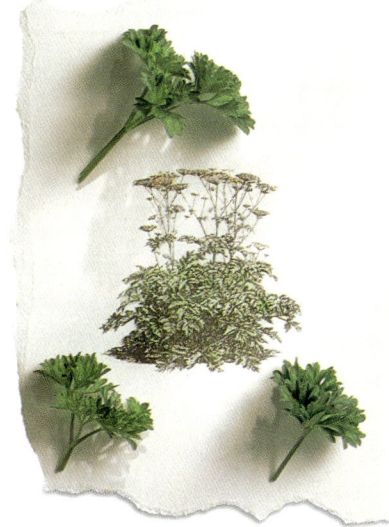

Parsley juice combined with honey can help to ease the irritation caused by bee stings.

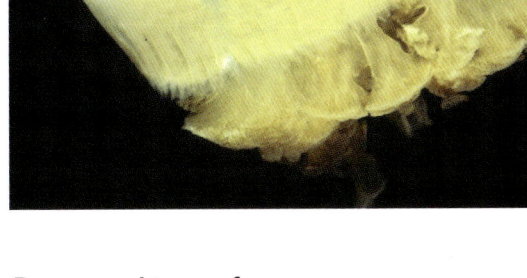

Remedies for Stinging Nettle Stings

Apply the juice from the stems of the nettles. Dock leaves, which often grow nearby, can also be wrapped around the affected area to ease the pain.

Remedies for Jellyfish Stings

Pour seawater over the affected area for ten minutes. The water releases the remaining toxins. Cold cider vinegar, ice, alcohol or diluted ammonia applied to the sting are all effective.

FIRST AID
Cuts and Grazes

Cuts and grazes have a habit of looking far worse than they really are, but once minor injuries are cleaned up there are several remedies which can be used to help. If a cut is bleeding profusely, elevate the injured part and press a clean cloth directly onto the wound. The most important thing with any cut or graze is to get the affected area as clean as possible before applying any covering.

Remedies for Cuts and Grazes

Wash cuts and grazes with diluted witch hazel to prevent infection. You can also use Friar's balsam or a few drops of calendula in warm water. If none of this is to hand, warm, soapy water with a few drops of lemon juice or a teaspoon of salt added will do the trick. If you are in a remote place, then plain saliva can be a great healer.

Parsley juice or heavy cream can be placed directly onto a wound and covered with a gauze dressing.

Crush up some parsley leaves and apply the juice directly onto a cut or graze.

Change it every two hours to make sure the wound is cleansed efficiently. Try washing the wound with the water from boiled parsnips and apply the warm pulp as a poultice.

Garlic acts as a marvelous natural antiseptic, so make up a mixture of crushed garlic and honey for a healing poultice and apply it directly to cuts and grazes. Use honey neat and cover with a bandage to prevent air or moisture penetrating the wound.

For a gravel graze, apply bread mixed with egg yolk and warm milk directly to the graze in order to gently draw out any small pieces of grit. Mash up raw avocado and cover with sterile gauze to prevent infection and promote healing.

Washing cuts and grazes with witch hazel can help to prevent infection.

Honey is particularly effective at drawing out the tiny pieces of gravel that tend to be found in children's cuts and grazes. Lemon is one of nature's most powerful astringents, so use it raw on cuts and grazes to stop bleeding. It will sting like mad but it really does the trick.

Drinking a cup of peppermint tea will immediately help to clot blood. It is particularly useful for nosebleeds.

Garlic wine made from chopped garlic steeped in white wine for several hours will cleanse and prevent infections in wounds and cuts.

In order to protect the area after cleaning, you should apply a paste of garlic and honey and cover with some fine gauze.

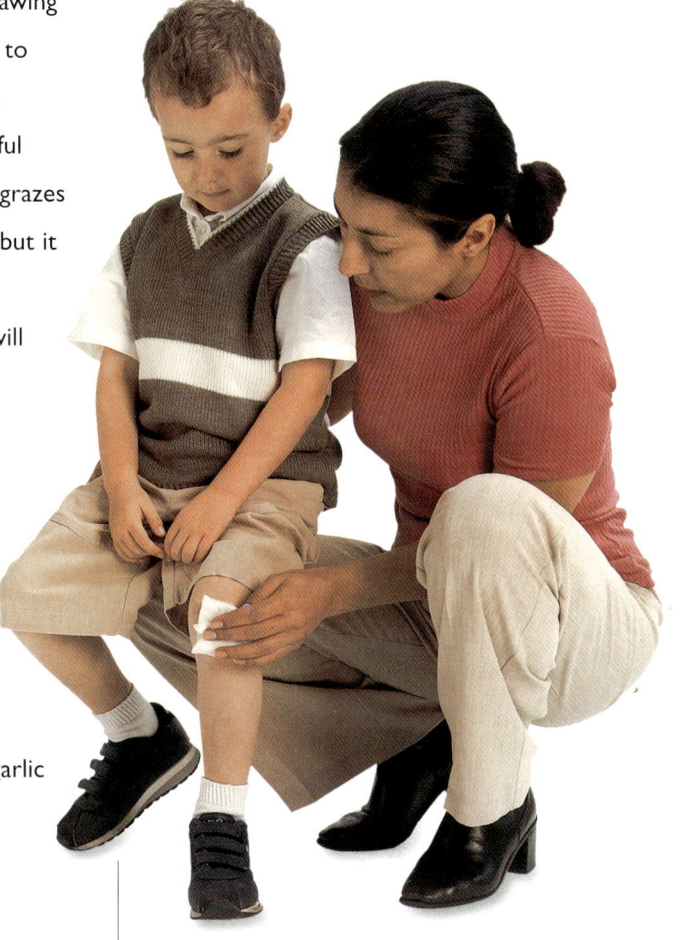

Apply a poultice of bread mixed with egg yolk and warm milk directly to a gravel graze to draw out any small pieces of grit.

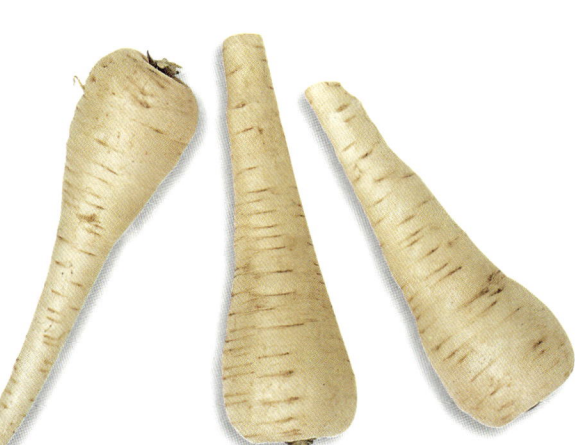

You can wash a wound with the water from boiled parsnips and apply the warm pulp as a poultice.

Washing Wounds

Use the following for washing wounds:

- Witch hazel (diluted)
- Friar's balsam (diluted)
- Calendula (diluted)
- Water with salt or drops of lemon juice
- Water in which parsnips have been boiled

FIRST AID
Bruises, Sprains, and Shock

Old wives used to recommend cold steak be placed directly onto a bruise. Nowadays, ice-cold water is the best cure, or a gentler method is to swab the bruise with a warm compress and massage it gently to stimulate the circulation. Injuries that cause bruises or sprains may lead to shock and even fainting, and caution is needed in these cases.

Remedies for Bruises and Sprains

If you have no ice, try a packet of frozen vegetables. Soak a sprained hand or foot in a bowl of warm water into which you have grated an onion and a potato.

Try a packet of frozen vegetables for bruises and sprains.

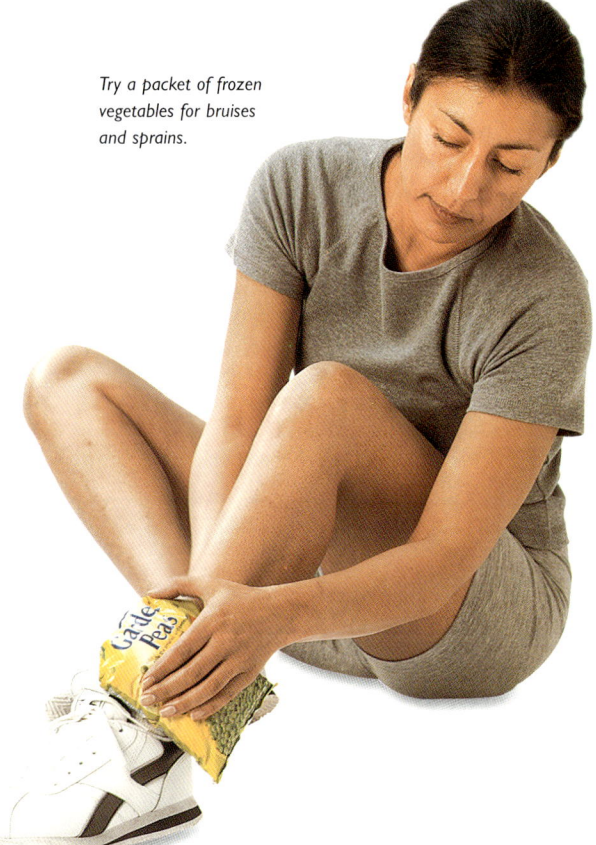

Massaging a bruise or sprain with onion will bring pain relief to the affected area.

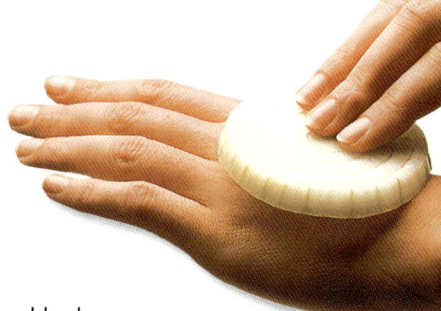

Half an onion rubbed on the affected area will quickly soothe it. Black eyes can be miraculously cured with a cold comfrey teabag placed directly over the offending area. Witch hazel will also help to soothe swellings and also to reduce inflammation and bleeding.

Apply hot or cold compresses of vinegar, particularly the type that is made from astringent fruits, such as raspberry, and rose, because they will help to reduce swelling and inflammation.

An old cook's remedy is parsley butter or oats mixed to a paste with boiling water and applied on a cloth to the affected area.

Remedies for Shock

Hot, sweet tea was always thought to be a restorative remedy for shock, and in fact honey added to any hot drink is a great healer. Basil and sage tea sweetened with honey is a great cure for someone who has experienced a mild shock.

Chamomile tea is also useful in this situation because it acts as a gentle sedative and therefore eases tension.

Orange blossom in hot water is believed to relieve anxiety. Not only can it be given to a patient as a kind of infusion, orange blossom water has a further point in its favor; a flannel can be steeped in the liquid to cool a patient down. Its soothing and refreshing properties will help to restore calm.

Cinnamon and honey dissolved in boiling water will help to pep someone up after they have fainted.

Remedies for Fainting

A hot tea made from peppermint, sage, lemon balm or rosemary will quickly revive someone coming round after fainting. Cinnamon and honey dissolved in boiling water are also good for this. Angelica was believed by ancient wise women to be the elixir of life and can be an excellent tonic.

Caution

- If you receive a blow to the head it may cause concussion, and you should always be seen by a doctor.

- Any injury that causes bruising or a sprain may also cause shock and fainting.

- There is a big difference between clinical shock, which can kill, and the sort of mild shock people suffer when they receive bad news or minor injuries. Again, it is best to seek medical advice.

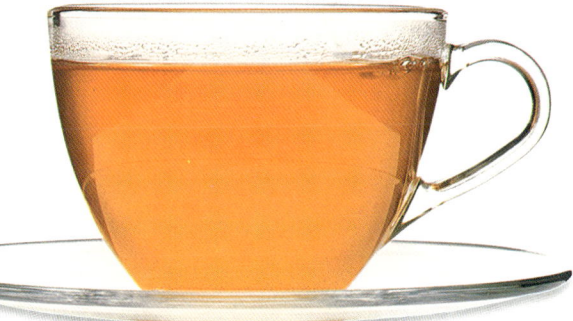

Chamomile tea and basil and sage tea are very effective means of restoring calm and will help in the management of shock.

GENERAL AILMENTS
Colds, Flu, and Coughs

Plenty of garlic or the herb echinacea will help boost the immune system and stop colds and flu from getting a hold. If you should be unlucky, however, at the first sign of a cold and fever make up a mustard footbath by adding one teaspoon of dried mustard to a bowl of very hot water. Mustard has a warming effect and inhaling an infusion will clear phlegm and draw infection and congestion away from the chest.

Remedies for Colds and Flu

Lemon and honey are traditional remedies for colds and flu—lemon because of its high vitamin C content and because it improves the body's ability to expel toxins, and honey because it can help to soothe a sore throat. You could make up a hot drink with the juice of two to four lemons and stir in a dessertspoon of honey for a comforting home remedy.

Add fresh ginger or peppermint, or their essential oils, to a hot bath or footbath. They both help you to perspire, which gets rid of toxins from the body. A ginger footbath also draws away blood from the head to the feet and in this way can reduce the heat congestion you so often feel in the rest of the body when you are suffering from a cold or flu.

Echinacea, available in tablet form, helps to boost the immune system and keep colds and flu at bay.

Garlic is a natural antibiotic and is good for all bronchial problems and lung complaints. If you eat garlic neat, try eating a sprig of parsley or dandelion leaf afterward to freshen your breath.

Onions are excellent for colds. Put a thick slice of onion into boiling water and add half a teaspoon of cayenne pepper. Strain and drink the liquid hot at bedtime.

Pour 2 cups of hot water over a handful of fresh pine needles, put a towel over your head and inhale the vapors deeply to counteract congestion.

You can even add a little lemon and

Garlic can act as a natural antibiotic and is good for all bronchial problems.

Pine needles can provide relief from chestiness. Pour hot water over some pine needles in a bowl, place a towel over your head and the bowl and inhale the vapors.

honey to the remaining water and drink it so that you increase your levels of vitamins C and A, which will help to speed up your recovery from illness.

Eat plenty of yogurt, which can kill bacteria on its own. It will also help your body to produce more antibodies that will kill any invading organisms.

Remedies for Coughs

If you have a persistent cough, try a poultice of roasted onion applied to the chest every two hours. Onions can also be drunk as a warm broth to cleanse the airways and to reduce congestion.

Try an infusion of grated fresh ginger root with spices such as cloves and cinnamon to help ease a chesty cough.

In Romany medicine, nettles are believed to rid the lungs and stomach of excess phlegm. For asthma and bronchitis, add a handful of young nettles to 1 cup of boiling water. Strain and drink the juice.

A cabbage leaf poultice works well when the chest is tight from coughing. Cabbage has an extraordinary ability to draw out toxins.

Crush the leaves with a rolling pin until the juice starts to appear. Place three or four leaves over the chest area and cover with gauze. Then place a warm blanket over to keep it in place. You can also drink the juice of the cabbage sweetened with a teaspoon of honey.

If you have a cold, you could try a bedtime drink of onion and cayenne pepper in hot water to soothe the symptoms.

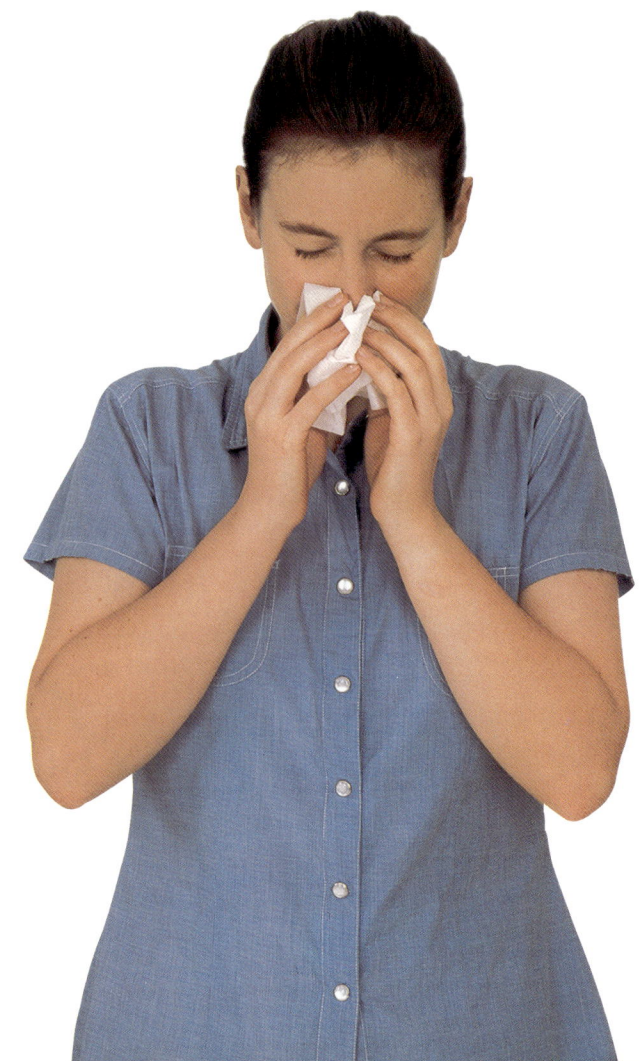

GENERAL AILMENTS
Sore Throat and Fever

At the first signs of a fever, lemon juice and honey or apple cider vinegar and honey diluted in plenty of warm water will help. Cold drinks of lemon juice, lemon barley water or fresh unsweetened fruit juices are all good remedies and will help to bring a temperature down.

Remedies for a Sore Throat

For a bad sore throat, make up a gargle with either salt, lemon juice or cider vinegar diluted with warm water. The salt helps to destroy the bacteria that cause the sore throat and helps to relieve the burning sensation. Squeeze the oil of a whole garlic clove into

Salt, lemon juice or cider vinegar in a glass of warm water makes an effective gargle to ease a sore throat.

Hyssop, a herb belonging to the mint family, can provide a boost to the immune system in the form of a tea or tisane.

a bowl, mix with cayenne pepper and warm salt water and soak a clean cloth in the liquid. Wear the cloth around your throat for instant relief. Gargling with plain salt water can also be soothing.

Echinacea acts as a natural antibiotic by boosting the body's immune system and fighting infection and illness. Garlic and onions relieve congestion and infections by reducing the amount of mucus in the nasal cavities.

Blackcurrants, crushed up in boiling water, can help your body to fight infection and inflammation.

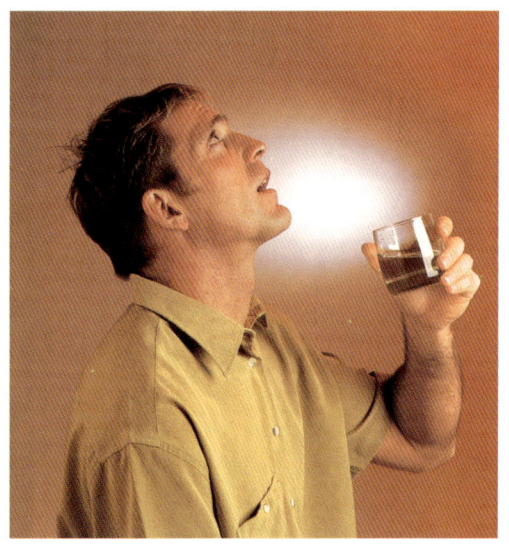

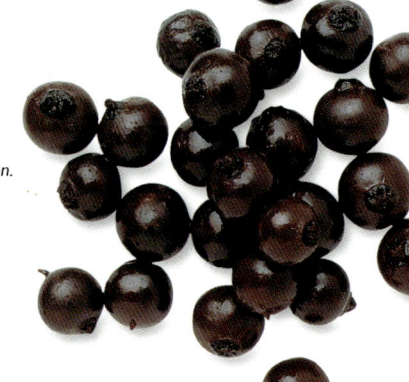

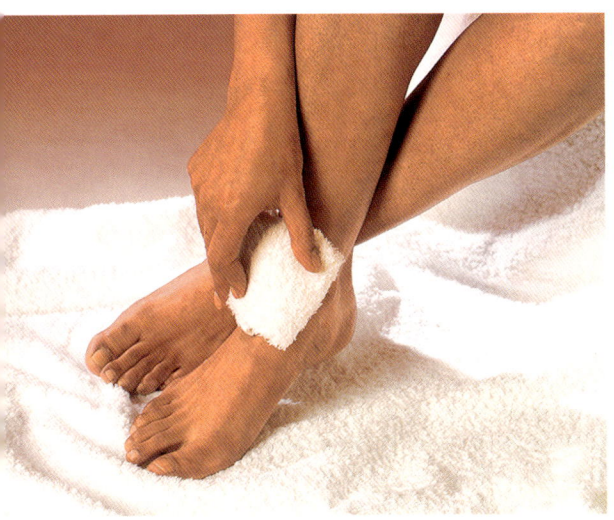

Try using a cool water compress applied to the legs and feet as a means of calming a fever.

Blackcurrants also counter infection and inflammation. Try a spoonful crushed into a cupful of boiling water and left to infuse for ten minutes—sip the drink slowly and chew the fruit. Red sage is the most famous remedy for sore throat—a tea made from the herb and drunk with a dash of cider vinegar will work wonders.

There is also a variety of teas and tisanes that help the immune system fight back. Some of the best remedies include hyssop, a member of the mint family. Lemon, which contains Vitamin C, and any tea that contains

Boil angelica root in water to bring down a fever. You might need to add lemon, honey, and brandy to make it more palatable.

Ancient Remedy for Fever

An ancient remedy for fever involved mixing cloves, cream of tartar and some cinnamon stick in a little tea with molasses or honey added. If you drank it every day of your life it was supposed to prevent fevers from occurring!

antioxidants will also help rid the body of free radicals which damage the cells in the body.

Remedies for Fever

You can calm a fever by applying cool water compresses to the legs and feet. Add some lavender or peppermint essential oils. Remove the compresses as soon as they warm up.

To combat infection you could use a cooled infusion of rosemary instead of cool water.

Angelica root boiled and infused in water will help to bring down a fever. Add the juice of two lemons, some honey and a drop of brandy to make it more palatable. Teas and tisanes that help to check a fever include hibiscus and basil.

For those with a cast-iron stomach, treat laryngitis with a syrup made up of grated horseradish root, lemon juice, and honey which has been left to stand in hot milk or water, then strained.

GENERAL AILMENTS
Hay Fever and Allergies

Hay fever is an allergy to the pollen released by grasses, flowers, and trees in spring and summer. The pollen causes cells to release histamine, which results in streaming eyes, runny nose, sneezing, and a sore itchy throat. Allergic reactions can also be caused by house-dust mites or the fur of animals or feathers of birds. Asthma is on the increase in the Western world—the jury is still out on the cause—but many people believe pollution to be a major factor.

Remedies for Hay Fever

In the old days people chewed natural honeycomb, which was supposed to protect them from allergies of every type. You can still find it in some health stores and it is worth a try. Eating plenty of garlic is also thought to counteract allergic reactions. Chamomile tea is a natural antihistamine—add honey to build up your immunity to pollen.

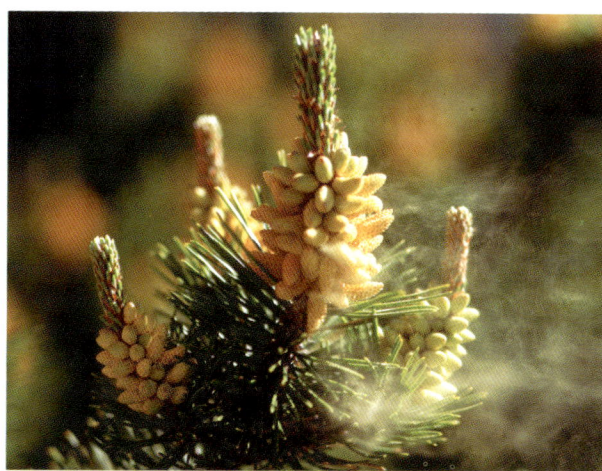

Pollen brings misery to many every year in the form of hay fever, which produces itchy eyes, runny nose, and sneezing.

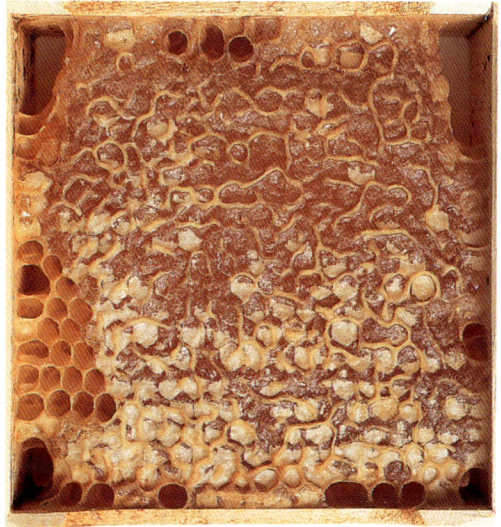

You could grate some horseradish and sniff it to help to clear out the sinuses as well as to stimulate breathing.

You could try taking a teaspoon of English mustard combined with a tablespoon of molasses first thing in the morning and last thing at night.

Natural honeycomb was once believed to protect people from all kinds of allergies.

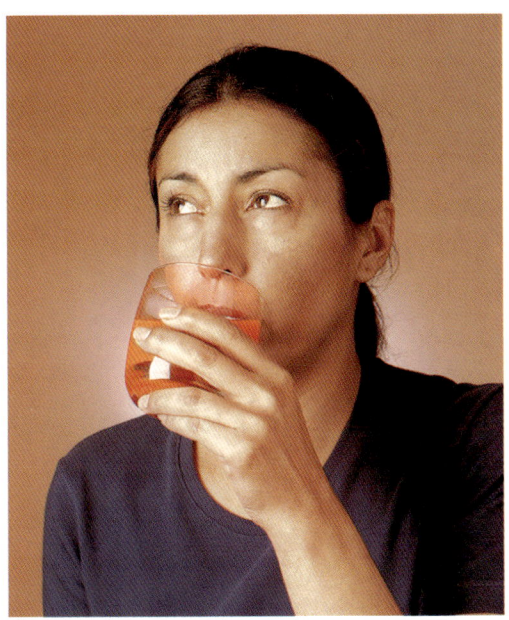

Fresh carrot juice is believed to help protect against asthma attacks. Drinking a glass a day could help to reduce the risk.

Elderflower tea or syrup drunk hot at bedtime will help keep the sniffles of hay fever at bay. Make your own syrup by mixing up elderflower heads, 2 cups of brown sugar, three lemons, and two sliced oranges. Add this to $7\frac{1}{2}$ cups of water and $\frac{1}{4}$ cup of tartaric acid. Steep it in a covered bowl for 24 hours, strain into a big pan and bring to a boil until the sugar is dissolved. Cool, then bottle or freeze, and drink as needed.

Garlic is useful for both hay fever and asthma. Chop it and add it raw to salads. A Russian remedy recommends inhaling an infusion of two or three cloves of crushed garlic added to a basin of hot water.

Remedies for Asthma

Nettles and onions can protect against asthma. Or try soaking a fresh cabbage leaf in hot water until saturated and drink the liquid. Chew two cloves of garlic a day or make up a drink from three heads of garlic, $2\frac{1}{2}$ cups of water, $1\frac{1}{4}$ cups of cider vinegar and a spoonful of honey. Simmer the garlic cloves in the water for half an hour, add the vinegar and honey and simmer until it forms a syrupy consistency. Drink a sherry-glassful each day. Drink a small glass of carrot juice daily to reduce the risk of asthma attacks.

Irish moss is a jelly, which you can get from some health food stores. Combine it with half an onion, two cloves of garlic and half a cup of honey to make a syrup. It can be taken every couple of hours or as needed.

Hay fever symptoms can be relieved by several natural home remedies, including elderflower tea.

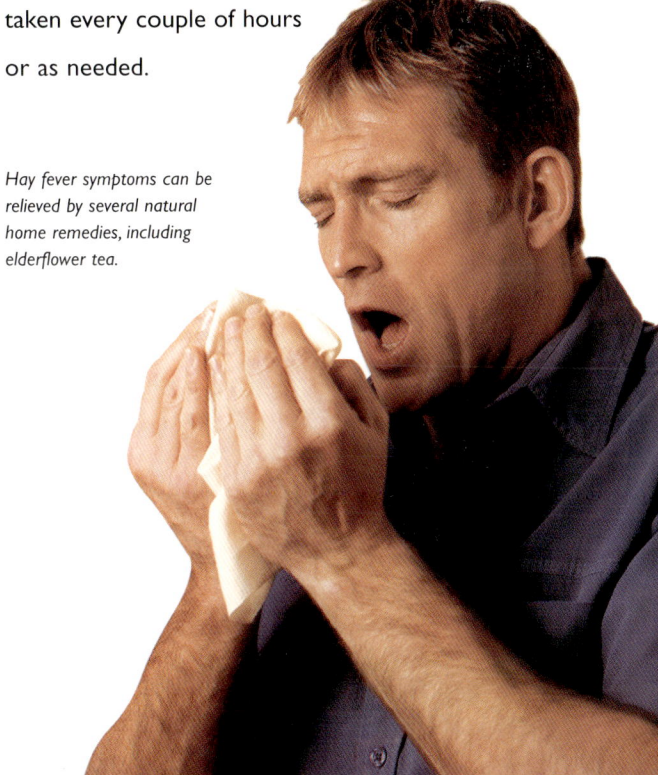

GENERAL AILMENTS
Back Pain

About 80% of us will have some form of back pain at some time in our lives. Many people suffer in silence for years because they know there simply is no cure. Rest and warmth provide some comfort, but there is also a variety of remedies, particularly poultices, that can be applied to ease the pain—even if only temporarily. With any sort of back pain it is always best to consult a doctor.

Remedies for Lumbago

Massage is an excellent remedy for most kinds of back problem. Make up a soothing massage oil from peppermint or cilantro oil in a tablespoon of almond oil. Massage it well into the muscles of the back.

Lumbago is a rheumatic pain in the lower region of the back and can be treated with similar remedies

Lumbago is rheumatic pain in the lower region of the back.

to those given for arthritis (see page 27). Some poultices may also be helpful. Cook up whole oats, then mash them with vinegar and apply them to the painful area as hot as possible.

Boil up cabbage leaves in milk until they become like jello, spread this mixture on the affected area with a cloth and leave it on overnight, covered with gauze held in place with plaster. This helps to release toxins from the body and, although it may not endear you to your bed partner, you will feel rested after a good night's sleep!

Shake together a cup of vinegar and turpentine and add a dessertspoon of powdered camphor and a whole egg. Keep the mixture refrigerated and use as a back rub when necessary.

Remedies for Sciatica

Sciatica is an excruciating back condition caused by pressure on the sciatic nerve which runs down the back of the leg to the knee.

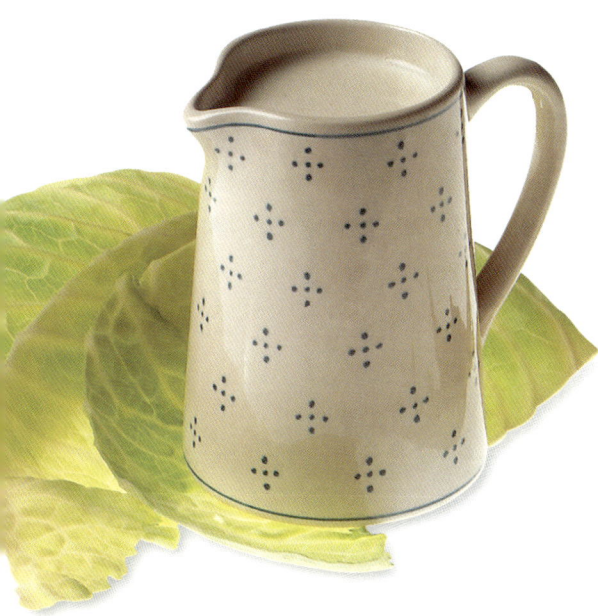

Cabbage leaves boiled up in milk turn into a kind of jello that can be applied to the back to ease the pain of lumbago.

will ease the pain of sciatica, particularly if it is brought on by cold and damp. A daily supplement of seaweed extract is invaluable for back pain of any sort because of its iodine content. A tablespoon of mustard or cayenne pepper in a hot bath will ease a bad back. You can also get relief from back pain by taking a warm bath infused with nettles and by having a lot of rest in a firm bed.

Make up a camphor rub from quarter of a teaspoon each of camphor and mustard powder. Add $1\frac{1}{4}$ cups of pure turpentine and $1\frac{1}{4}$ cups of sunflower oil, mix with $1\frac{1}{4}$ cups of rubbing alcohol and shake the ingredients together. Use it to massage an aching back or any other limbs that are seized up. Keep the area warm.

It is caused by pressure in the lower spine, inflammation of the nerve itself or by back strain or injury, which may need to be seen by a back expert.

Some people swear by ivy. Take two handfuls of ivy, chop well and mix with two handfuls of bran. Stir to a paste with $1\frac{1}{4}$ cups of water and warm over a low heat for 10 minutes. Apply to the affected area using a cloth and leave for half an hour.

A cupful of Epsom salts added to a hot bath

Ivy leaf is believed to make an excellent remedy for sciatica.

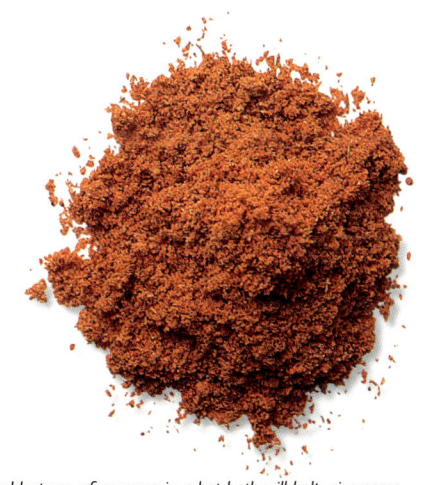

A tablespoon of cayenne in a hot bath will help give some relief from most back problems.

GENERAL AILMENTS
Rheumatism and Arthritis

Arthritis affects the joints and bones and can be an extremely painful and debilitating condition. Rheumatism describes the swelling, soreness, stiffness, and aching of joints and includes rheumatic fever and bursitis, a painful condition resulting from inflammation of the bursa, the fluid-filled sacs that cushion the joints.

Remedies for Rheumatism

Chilies and bell peppers are rich in capsaicin, an active chemical that desensitizes nerves and controls pain. The Mayna Jivaro tribe of Peru still apply chili fruits directly to their teeth to cure toothache, and this has prompted Western doctors to run trials to see if it may work as a pain reliever for rheumatic diseases.

Native Americans used to swear by a poultice of sage, tobacco, angelica, and balsam

Bell peppers contain a lot of capsaicin, a chemical that can control pain.

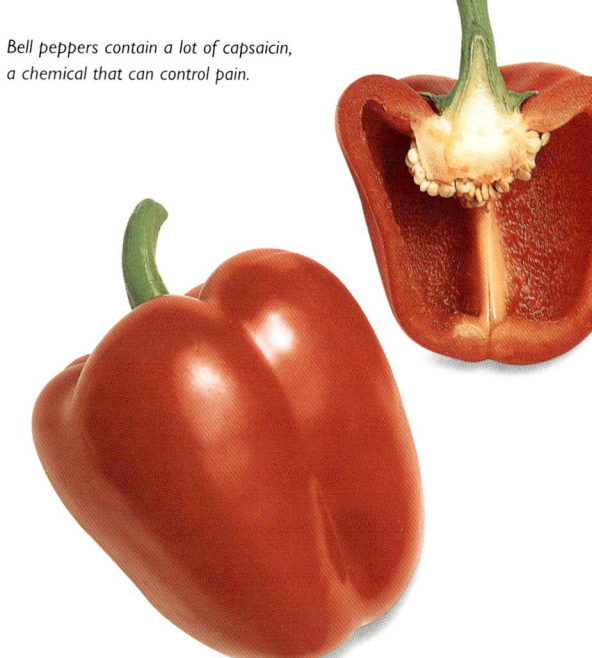

Yogurt with grated apple and raw oats can help to reduce joint pain.

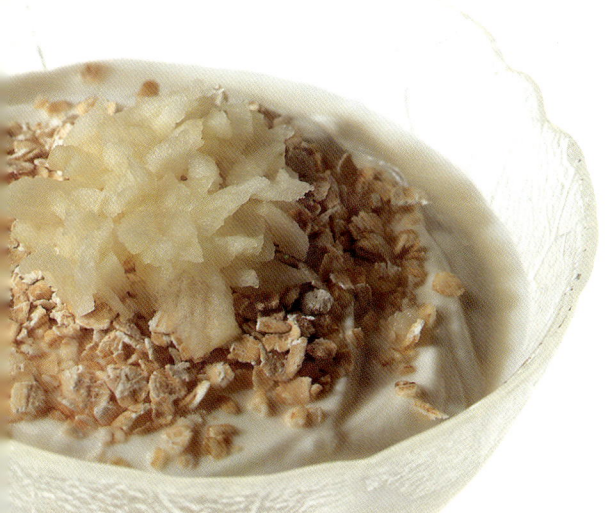

for rheumatic aches and pains. A less dramatic remedy is Epsom salts added to a hot bath, which will ease the pain, or try mixing a scant tablespoon of dried mustard or cayenne pepper into your bathwater.

Eat plenty of onions and garlic—you can even make up a delicious onion drink by chopping up three unpeeled onions and boiling them gently in $2\frac{1}{2}$ cups of water.

Garlic pounded in olive oil with parsley and eaten on whole-wheat bread has been known to help, or a breakfast of grated apple with raw oats and yogurt is also good.

Potatoes can provide pain relief for arthritis sufferers.

Remedies for Arthritis

Turmeric is a well-known cure for arthritis, so use plenty in your food. Drink warm milk with a teaspoon of ground turmeric mixed in three times a day. A back rub made from a scant tablespoon of cayenne pepper in a cup of olive oil and applied to inflamed joints will bring a soothing heat to the aching area. Boil $2\frac{1}{2}$ cups of apple cider vinegar with a scant tablespoon of cayenne pepper, cool and use as a compress on the affected area. Cayenne can cause skin irritation, so make sure it heats the area but does not cause burning.

A good preventative measure is to mix a teaspoon of cider vinegar and honey in hot water and drink it first thing in the morning. Or try drinking the juice of one lemon in hot water sweetened with honey before breakfast.

Nettle soup, which is made with fresh nettle tops, chopped onion and garlic, or plain nettle tea, are both tried and tested remedies for arthritis.

Potatoes have excellent anti-inflammatory properties and can relieve pain. To make a potato poultice, boil three large potatoes in their skins until tender. Place them in some cheesecloth and mash. Apply the sack to the affected area. Remove it only once it has cooled down completely.

Remedies for Bursitis

Make a poultice of cooked cabbage leaves, mashed and applied warm between layers of gauze or cheesecloth. Linseed, marshmallow, and slippery elm are other comforting herbs that can be taken as supplements. Boil up hot apple cider vinegar with cayenne pepper and apply as a compress, as for arthritis.

Turmeric can be used in many dishes and even drunk added to warm milk to counter the pain of arthritis.

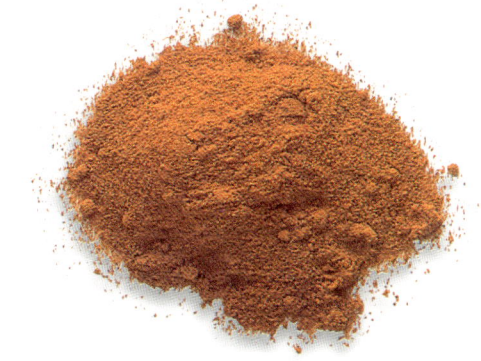

GENERAL AILMENTS
Hangovers

The best way to avoid a hangover is to avoid too much alcohol! However, that is little consolation if you are suffering the agonies of a banging head, parched throat, and the constant threat of being sick. If you know you have drunk too much, you can prevent a hangover by drinking at least 5 cups of water before going to bed. This will help to flush out some of the toxins. Colas and sodas can also help your throbbing head because they alkalize the acid in the stomach.

Remedies for Hangovers

For some reason, eggs have always been a big feature of hangover cures across all cultures. And, in fact, eggs do contain a certain chemical now known to neutralize the effects of alcohol, so it seems that the old eggnog remedy or fried eggs the morning after may work well after all!

For an upset stomach or nausea, try grating some fresh ginger root into a mug of boiling water and sipping it slowly.

Colas and sodas alkalize the acid in the stomach and help to stop the banging sensation in your head.

Tea made from fresh ginger will soothe a queasy stomach when you have drunk too much the night before.

Drinking ginger tea will also soothe your stomach, and it tastes delicious, too.

Umeboshi plums, available at Asian markets and health food stores, have long been reputed to cure hangovers. They may make some people want to vomit, but those people who have managed to keep them down swear by them.

One of the best herbal fixits for a hangover is peppermint tea. Adding organic honey will also ease your headache and begin the process of rehydration.

Replenish your lost vitamin C with a glass of fresh orange juice and add a teaspoon of lime juice or a dash of cumin powder to really get you back in gear. Drinking a cup of thyme

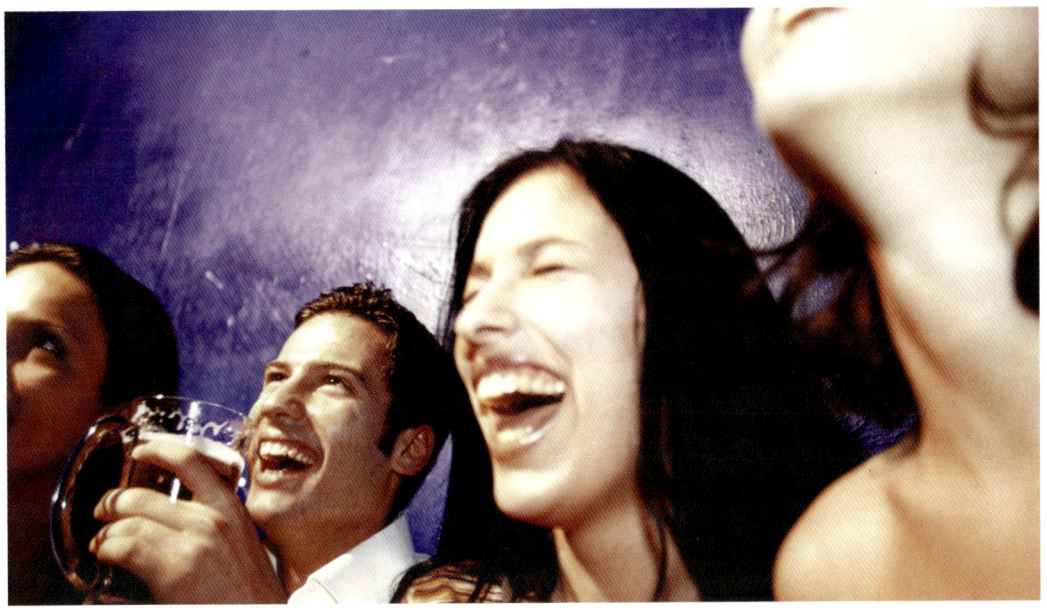

Eat, drink, and be merry! But be prepared for the morning after the night before and have a natural hangover remedy to hand.

tea will ease your headache and queasy stomach more effectively and safely than many over-the-counter pain relievers.

Try the hair of the dog! Peel a whole head of garlic and put in a pan with 1½ cups of red wine. Bring to a boil and simmer for 20 minutes. Strain and drink slowly. It is the tannins, not the alcohol, that help to cure your banging head!

Once you can face food again, a vegetable broth which is high in potassium and natural minerals will help to replace lost fluids and minerals. Make it from celery stalks, zucchini, beets or carrots. Try to avoid sulfur-containing vegetables such as broccoli, onions, and cabbage. Replace intestinal flora with good bacteria from live yogurt.

Try a soothing bath with essential oils of eucalyptus, peppermint, and sandalwood. A cup of peppermint tea will also help if you are feeling queasy. Soak a towel in ice-cold water and wrap it around your forehead. The coldness should help to shrink away your headache.

Cook a healthy broth using vegetables to replace lost minerals and fluids.

GENERAL AILMENTS
Stomach Troubles

Indigestion is often known as heartburn, and as its name suggests it causes a feeling of discomfort just below the breastbone around the heart area. Eating too much, too quickly, is the main cause of indigestion, with symptoms varying from wind and rumblings in the stomach to pain or nausea.

Remedies for Indigestion

Ripe bananas are natural antacids and can soothe an inflamed stomach. If none is available, try cider vinegar or lemon juice in hot water, which alkalizes an acid stomach. Ginger tea, made from fresh ginger root if possible, also warms and soothes an acid stomach. Drink an infusion

Infuse fresh mint and drink sweetened with honey for nausea.

of hot peppermint tea or try teas such as fennel, lemon balm, or cinnamon. Slippery elm powder dissolved in hot water gives immediate relief.

Mix two tablespoons of baking soda with one teaspoon of ground ginger in cold water and drink before sitting down to breakfast to prevent indigestion.

Tea made from peppermint helps combat feelings of nausea.

Remedies for Nausea

Peppermint is considered to be an excellent cure for nausea. Although it has long been associated with the relief of indigestion and travel sickness, how it works is little understood. It is believed to work by relaxing the

Water

- Avoid drinking water with a meal because it dilutes the gastric acid and leads to incomplete digestion.
- Water can also cause the fats and oils in the food to cling together, which stops them being absorbed properly.
- Drink water ten minutes before or three hours after eating.

esophageal sphincter and equalizing gastric pressures. Buy readymade peppermint tea bags or put four drops of peppermint oil, found with the cookery ingredients in the grocery store, in some hot water and let it cool. Drink slowly for quick relief from nausea. Infuse some fresh mint and drink sweetened with honey.

Remedies for Food Poisoning

Food poisoning can cause terrible vomiting, diarrhea and stomach cramps. It is the body's way of getting rid of food that is bad or disagrees with it and is usually caused by germs that inflame the lining of the stomach and intestines. The main problem

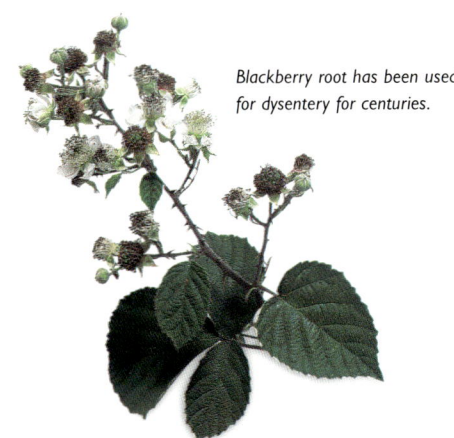

Blackberry root has been used for dysentery for centuries.

with food poisoning is fluid loss which causes dehydration, so it is important to keep up your liquid intake.

In the old days, remedies included a disgusting concoction of salt swiftly followed by a spoonful of castor oil. For mild food poisoning take raw garlic, which helps to fight the infection in the gut. Replace lost fluid by drinking plain water or diluted fruit juice.

Blackberry root has been used for years to combat the deadly form of dysentery so common in hot climates. During the American Revolution both sides accepted truces so that troops could go "rooting" for blackberry roots and leaves. It is still one of the safest remedies for children's diarrhea.

Stewed fennel, horseradish leaves or a strong dose of apple cider vinegar have all been used to help remove bad food from the digestive system.

Ripe bananas are believed to be natural antacids. They can provide relief from inflammation of the stomach.

GENERAL AILMENTS
Cystitis and Bladder Conditions

Cystitis is a painful condition caused by inflammation of the bladder. Symptoms include pain in the lower back and a stabbing pain when urinating. It is important to seek your doctor's advice if you have cystitis for any length of time, because if it continues it can lead to kidney infection. Cystitis has been called the "honeymoon disease" because it often occurs after sex. Drinking water and urinating as soon after sex as possible may help to prevent an attack.

Remedies for Cystitis

Plain water flushes out the kidneys better than anything and will help to get rid of the bacteria that are causing the infection. Drink plenty and often. Make up $2\frac{1}{4}$ cups of mild chamomile tea and drink it throughout the day to flush germs out of the bladder.

Try one teaspoon of baking soda in a glass of tepid water every three hours. It makes the urine less acidic, which stops bacteria from breeding—it also relieves the burning sensation that so often accompanies cystitis.

Apply live yogurt to the affected area—its friendly bacteria can help to fight invading germs. Make up some homemade barley water by boiling up a cupful of barley in enough water to cover it. Add the zest of a lemon and simmer until the barley is soft. Strain off the barley, add some honey and sip slowly throughout the day.

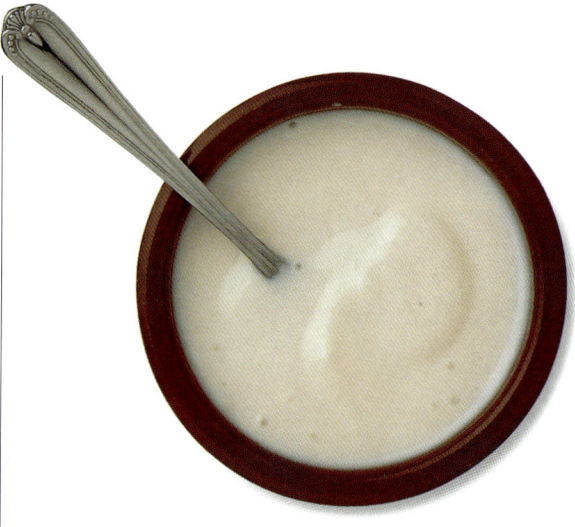

Plain live yogurt is a traditional natural home remedy used to combat the discomfort of cystitis.

Cranberry juice can reach the parts that other juices can't reach. A substance in cranberries appears to prevent bacteria from sticking to the walls of the urinary tract where they would normally proliferate. When you drink cranberry juice the bacteria lose their grip and are washed away.

Cranberry juice is a well-known cure for cystitis.

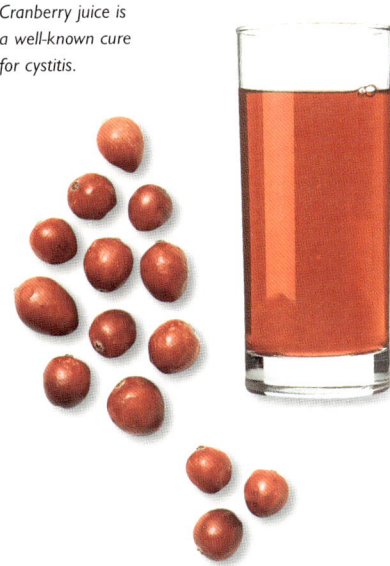

Make an onion soup from three or four onions steeped in 4¼ cups of hot water. Drink it throughout the day—it tastes disgusting but does the trick. Horseradish also stimulates digestion and encourages the kidneys to flush through urine. Horseradish can be grated into foods or boiled up with mustard seed and water as a drink.

Experts now believe the same component may also be present in blueberries. Eat the berries or pulp them with a little water in a food processor.

Turnips, celery stalk, fennel, and onions are all good diuretics; so are dandelion roots and stinging nettle leaves. Add any of these raw to salads.

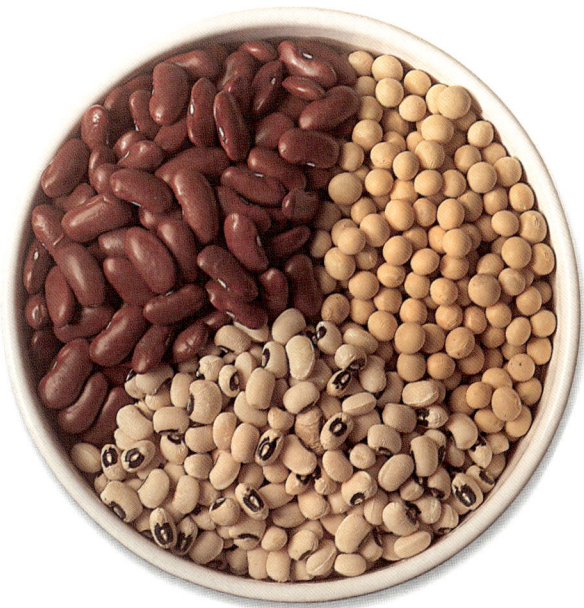

Kidney beans, soya beans, and black-eyed beans can make an appetizing dish which really benefits the kidneys.

Onions are a good diuretic, and can be added to many different dishes, including soups and salads.

Kidney beans are also helpful for any kidney or urinary tract infections. You can also try black soybeans or black-eye peas. Cook them with garlic and use them to replace meat in the diet. Chinese herbalists swear by seaweed, fenugreek, and saw palmetto for good results.

GENERAL AILMENTS
Bowel Problems

Constipation, diarrhea, irritable bowel syndrome (IBS), and hemorrhoids are four of the most debilitating conditions known to humankind—made all the worse because nobody wants to talk about them. Constipation occurs for many reasons, the most common of which is poor bowel habits learned from a young age, and can lead to hemorrhoids. Medications including antidepressants can also cause constipation. Diarrhea is often the result of food poisoning, and either constipation or diarrhea can be symptoms of IBS.

Remedies for Constipation

Anyone who remembers syrup of figs from their childhood will not be at all surprised to learn that both figs and prunes are well-known laxatives.

Drinking cooked cabbage or carrot juice can also help to ease constipation, or you could mash up raw apricots with a little honey in a bowl of yogurt.

Rhubarb stewed with honey will also have the desired effect. Strawberries have a mild

Figs and prunes are effective laxatives and can help to ease the discomfort of constipation.

laxative effect and are particularly useful when constipation is due to excessive meat or fat in the diet.

Remedies for Diarrhea

Rice pudding is one of the oldest remedies for diarrhea. Make your own with $1\frac{1}{2}$ cups of milk, a pinch of salt, a scant cup of brown sugar, a teaspoon of vanilla extract, two to four eggs, grated lemon zest and 2 cups of cooked white rice. Add all the ingredients together and mix well. Spread the mixture in a buttered baking dish and cook for an hour. Sprinkle with cinnamon.

Boil rice in water for one and a half hours, then strain and drink the liquid to soothe an

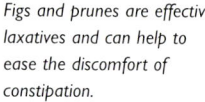

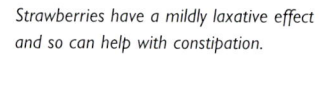

Strawberries have a mildly laxative effect and so can help with constipation.

Try grated apple that has gone brown—the oxidized pectin acts like an over-the-counter medicine to cure diarrhea.

irritated bowel. You could also make a thick oatmeal drink by cooking together 1 cup of oats and 5 cups of water for five minutes. Strain and drink frequently. Oats also have a calming effect on the bowel, and starchy fluids tend to stop vomiting and reduce fluid loss.

Add a teaspoon of cornstarch to a glass of water at room temperature—it tastes disgusting, so drink it quickly Repeat the dose every three or four hours.

Blueberries contain compounds called anthocyanosides which control diarrhea, so add them to your breakfast cereal.

Try eating a grated apple which has been allowed to go brown. The pectin oxidizes and acts like many proprietary brands of diarrhea remedies—slightly unripe bananas have the same effect.

Remedies for IBS

Peppermint has a well proven anti-spasmodic effect on the smooth muscle of the intestines—drink peppermint tea or, if you have mint growing in your yard, chew the fresh

leaves or sprinkle them on salads. Potatoes can reduce stomach acid because they contain small amounts of atropine which has an anti-spasmodic effect. Wash and dice a large potato and steep it overnight in a cup of cold water with salt. Strain and drink the water every morning on an empty stomach. A two-day diet of potatoes will flush out toxins and waste from the body and help to purify the blood.

Remedy for Hemorrhoids

Rub a small amount of either witch hazel or lemon juice into the affected area with a cotton wool swab before going to bed.

Rice pudding is one of the oldest remedies for diarrhea.

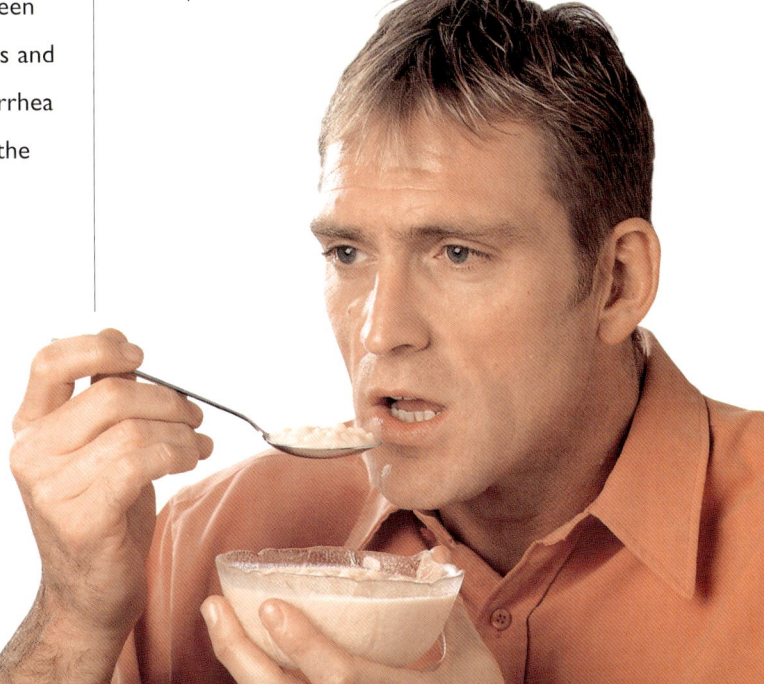

GENERAL AILMENTS
Skin Problems

Skin problems often reflect what is happening inside the body. Acne normally appears at adolescence and is believed to be caused by hormonal imbalances which produce too much of the oily substance in the skin known as sebum. Psoriasis occurs when skin cells reproduce up to a hundred times faster than normal. The skin then builds up in dry, flaky patches and causes itching and irritation.

Remedies for Acne

Avocado may be rich in fatty oils but it also contains plenty of vitamins A, B complex, C, and E, which are all essential for good skin. It has strong anti-bacterial and anti-fungal properties, so it is excellent for acne or any other irritating skin conditions. Make up a paste of avocado pulp and apply to any dry skin rashes to soothe and moisturize.

Grate some horseradish, which is rich in sulfur, and infuse it in hot milk for half an hour. Strain it and use the liquid as a face wash. You can also

Avocados contain all the vitamins—A, B complex, C, and E—needed for a healthy skin.

leave a teaspoon of the grated root to dissolve in a cupful of cider vinegar for a week and use it in the same way. It will sting badly but works well.

Remedies for Eczema

Make a paste from a teaspoon of powdered marshmallow root or slippery elm mixed with hot water. Spread it onto the affected area and leave for 20 minutes, then wash off with an infusion of comfrey. Comfrey leaves also make a wonderful facial wash and will promote growth of new tissue.

Make a rice-flour poultice and apply it hot to the affected area. Eat plenty of asparagus, which helps promote the elimination of toxins through urine and is also considered a liver

Eating a grapefruit a day is a routine that can help relieve the symptoms of psoriasis.

Comfrey leaves can be turned into a marvelous facial wash for those affected by eczema.

tonic because of its high amino acid content. Drink the water of the asparagus after it has been steamed.

Beets were used by the Romans to relieve fever, but also stimulate the immune system and help to clear the blood. Drink the juice of cabbage, which contains anti-bacterial properties, to promote healing, and eat plenty of watercress, which contains sulfur.

Dandelions are a fantastic detoxifier of the liver, kidneys, blood, and tissues. Use a tincture of dandelion roots for eczema or acne.

Remedies for Psoriasis

Make up an anti-fungal herbal tea from hops. Eat a grapefruit a day for breakfast. Drink cranberry juice, eat prunes and plums, and avoid alcohol and smoking.

Make up a dandelion wine from a bunch of dandelion petals, 22 cups of water, two

oranges, and two lemons, cut into pieces, a pinch of yeast and 3lb of sugar. Boil the dandelion petals for 20 minutes and pour over the orange and lemon pieces. Allow the mixture to cool, then add the yeast and let stand for 48 hours. Strain the mixture through cheesecloth and pour into a pitcher. Let the wine stand for about six weeks before bottling. Keep for at least six months before drinking.

Eating plenty of watercress, which contains sulfur, is recommended as a treatment for eczema.

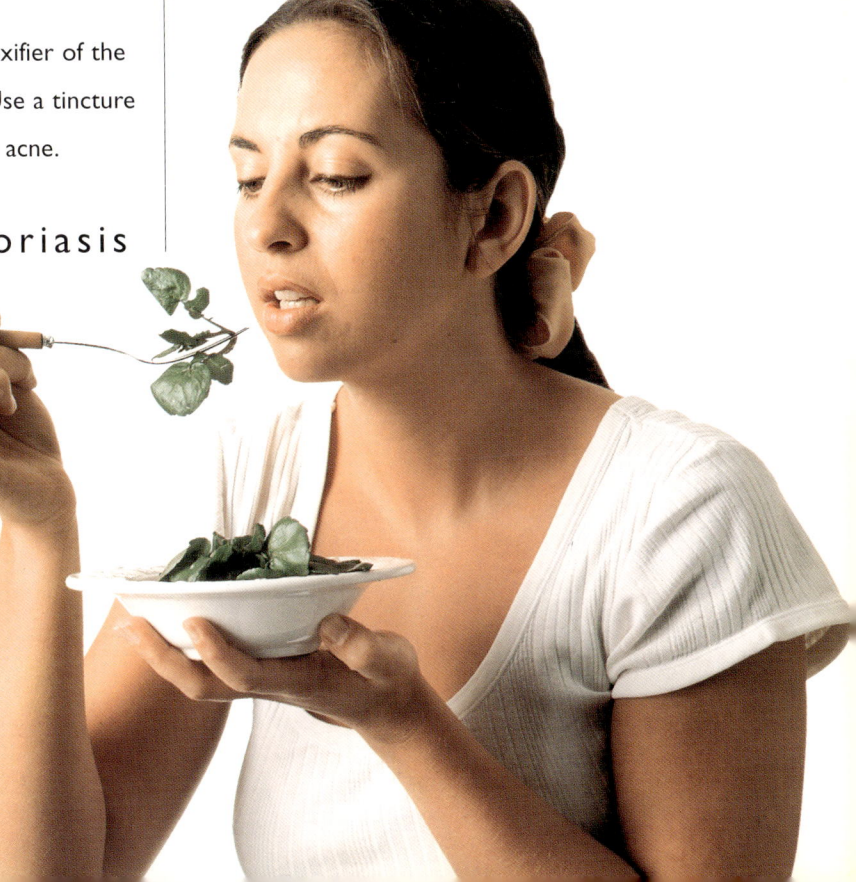

Toothache and Gum Disease

Unfortunately, toothache is an all-too-familiar condition in the Western world, and it is usually the result of poor care of the teeth and gums. Halitosis (bad breath) is often caused by sore gums or abscesses in the mouth.

Remedies for Toothache

Oil of cloves or a dried clove rubbed onto the gum around an aching tooth will help soothe it. Try chewing a clove over the offending tooth for instant relief, or pack dried hops or fresh peppermint into the tooth.

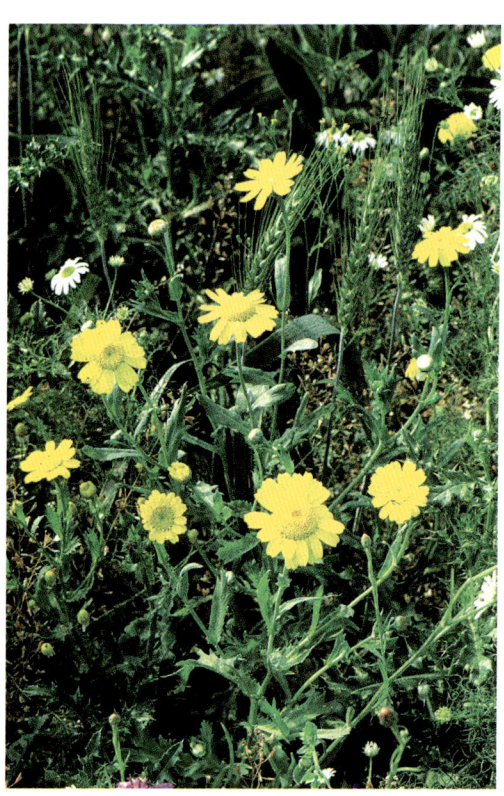

Raw cloves rubbed onto the offending tooth can cure a toothache, or chew one whole to find instant relief.

In Germany, dentists use a clove-based anesthetic to eradicate the pain of toothache. Native Americans used to apply the mashed green leaves or root of the willow as a poultice for toothache. You could make a mouthwash of vinegar and salt to ease the pain. Apply ground black pepper and fresh ginger to a piece of gauze and pack the tooth with it.

If you are not worried about being antisocial, you could plug a cavity with cotton wool soaked in onion or garlic juice. It will disinfect the whole area and give some relief from the pain.

You could try putting a slice of lightly boiled apple between the teeth to help to relieve the pain of toothache.

You can make a tincture of marigold that will help to ease the pain of a bad tooth or sore gums.

Remedies for Sore Gums

Cabbage is known for its anti-inflammatory properties, so you could dab a little white cabbage juice onto mouth sores.

Sore gums may be the result of vitamin B and C deficiency, so strengthen your gums by drinking plenty of rose hip or blackcurrant tea and tisanes.

Soak a small pad of cotton wool in tincture of marigold and press it to the sore gum or bad tooth.

Make a mouthwash out of marigold or agrimony, boiled in water and left to cool.

A tincture of lavender leaves rubbed onto the gums acts as an excellent antiseptic, or you could gargle with a cooled infusion of lavender leaves mixed with honey.

You can make your own natural toothpowder by mixing two parts of baking of soda to one part salt. If you have none to hand, you could even try cleaning your teeth with raw lemon.

Tincture of lavender leaves rubbed on the gum acts as an antiseptic.

Blueberries are astringent and antiseptic and are therefore good for combating mouth ulcers and gum infection.

Remedies for Mouth Ulcers

Eat plenty of blueberries—they are astringent and act as a strong antiseptic, and so they can be useful for mouth ulcers or sores and infections of the gums.

Try mixing two teaspoons of sea salt and two teaspoons of hydrogen peroxide in a large glass of warm water as a mouthwash. (NB: Don't swallow.) Hot salt water held in the mouth over an abscess also helps to disperse it.

Mouth Fresheners

- Try chewing on a few sprigs of parsley to freshen the mouth.
- Crush cloves in a cupful of boiling water, cool for five minutes and then use as a mouthwash.

Migraine and Headache

Most people experience headaches at some time or another. Some are caused by tension or stress, others are the result of too much alcohol or may herald a cold or flu. Migraine is more than just a serious headache. It is actually a neurological disorder which includes a pounding headache along with visual disturbance, nausea, and vomiting. If you have a headache that persists for any length of time, see a doctor.

Remedies for Headache

A warm cabbage leaf compress placed on the head can help to ease a headache, or try eating a crust of stale brown bread with butter and marmalade—a curious remedy, but very effective! A poultice of cucumber or raw potatoes placed on the brow can relieve a headache caused by too much sun.

Lavender will help to refresh and clear your head. You can make up your own

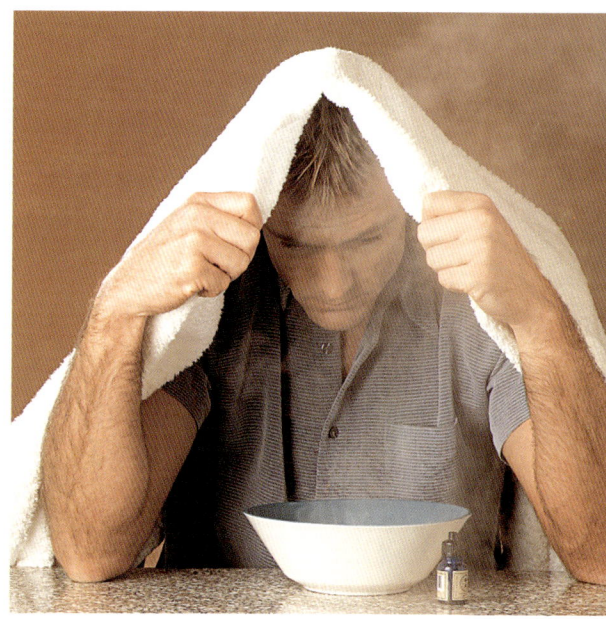

Apply a poultice of raw cucumber or raw potatoes to your brow to ease headaches.

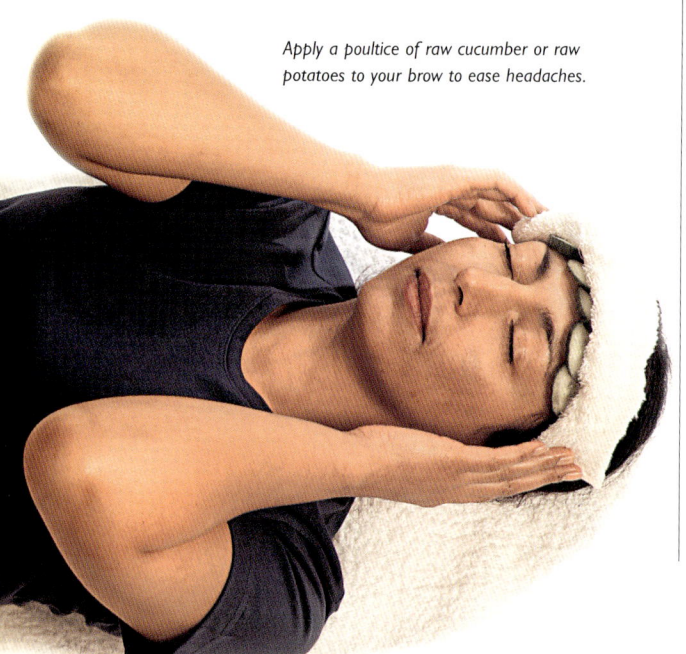

Steam inhalation is the best cure for a sinus headache. You can add various essential oils to help increase its efficacy.

lavender water with two tablespoons of dried lavender, two teaspoons of cinnamon, a pinch of grated nutmeg, and $4\frac{1}{4}$ cups of surgical spirit. Breathe in the delicious fumes for instant relief. Headaches caused by hypertension can also be eased by eating garlic, which lowers blood pressure.

Remedies for Sinus Headache

Sinus headaches respond best to steam inhalations. Add the essential oils of pine, eucalyptus, rosemary or thyme, either on their own or in combination. Apply a hot compress of plain water to the forehead. You can also infuse the water with lavender or peppermint oils. Lie down and breathe in the aroma, keeping the compress hot.

Remedies for Migraine

Feverfew is the main herb proven to have an effect on migraine. Oregano has also been reported to be effective—the dried leaf can be used as snuff to clear a blocked head, or simmer the fresh leaf in olive oil and use it to massage the temples.

A drink made from fresh ginger root has been shown to be almost as effective at preventing migraines (when taken daily) as powerful prescription drugs.

Add ginger oil to almond oil and massage onto the temples during early warning signs. Or try soaking your feet in a footbath which has either fresh ginger or peppermint added, or their essential oil. The bath will draw the blood away from

The herb feverfew has been proven in clinical trials to have an effect on migraine.

the head to the heat and provide some relief.

Eating a bowl of canned tomatoes simmered with basil and served with a dash of vinegar has been known to help migraine.

Make up an ointment out of oregano oil and petroleum jelly and smooth onto the temples.

If you can get hold of feverfew, make up a tea from the herb. If not, try peppermint and rosemary. Use two parts peppermint leaves and one part rosemary and let them steep in a mug of hot water for at least ten minutes.

A crust of stale brown bread spread with butter and marmalade seems to work for headaches.

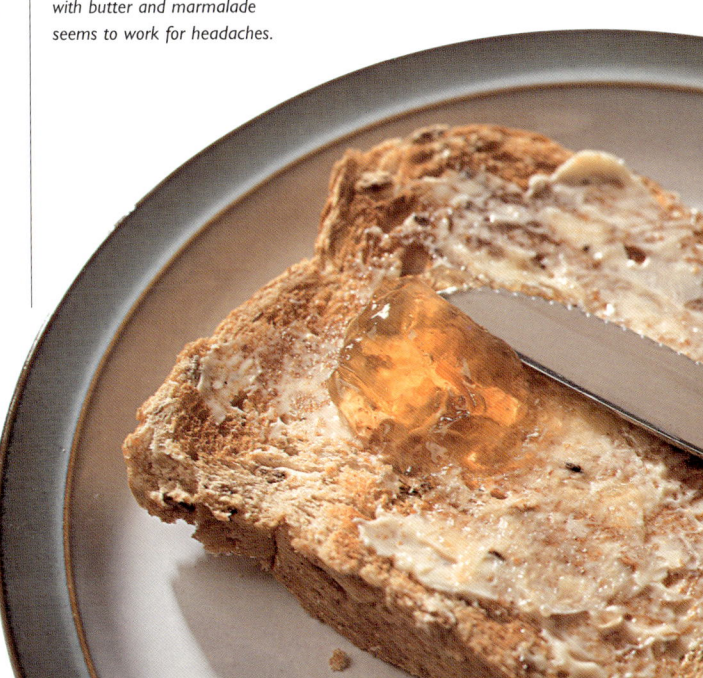

Earache and Neuralgia

Earache can be caused by a variety of things, from colds and catarrh to enlarged adenoids or an infection of the inner ear. Most home remedies are based on warmth and oil, but you should never poke the ear, no matter how bad the pain.

Any inflammation of the trigeminal nerve, which carries sensations into the skull near the ear, produces an excruciating spasmodic pain in one side of the face known as neuralgia. At one time, grated horseradish would have been applied to the

A lump of salt rolled in a hot, damp cloth and held against the ear can relieve earache.

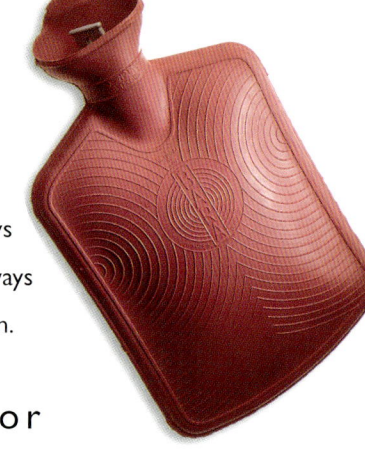

A hot water bottle wrapped in an old sweater can help soothe earache or neuralgia.

cheek until the pain subsided, but nowadays there are less harsh ways of curing the condition.

Remedies for Earache

Many earaches result from colds, flu or other types of congestion. If this is the case, you can reduce the mucus and phlegm with a tea made from elderflowers or a cold elderberry drink.

One of the best remedies for earache is a hot water bottle covered in a warm sweater and held close to the ear. Put a few drops of warm olive oil in the ear and lie on the opposite side for about five minutes while the oil flows down into the inner ear.

Crush a clove of garlic and let it rest in some warm olive oil for fifteen minutes, then strain the liquid. Soak a cotton wool ball in the liquid and place it just inside the outer earlobe.

Garlic, crushed, and soaked in olive oil, can be an effective means of countering infection in the ear.

The garlic combats infection. In the old days, a boiled onion placed on the affected ear was supposed to be a marvelous cure. Some used the juice of the onion in a warm oil.

You could also heat a teaspoon of almond oil and pour gently into the ear, then plug with a piece of cotton wool.

As a compress, try a lump of salt rolled in a cloth, steeped in hot water and wrung out, or a baked potato wrapped in wool—use both remedies as hot as you can stand it for the best effect.

Drink plantain tea to tone up the delicate membranes of the inner ear and prevent dizziness from ear inflammations.

Remedies for Neuralgia

Massage the gums right at the back of the mouth with a clove. Sleeping with a hop pillow has been known to cure this most painful of conditions, or try holding a hot poultice of porridge oats wrapped in cheesecloth against the area. Eating oats can also act as a stress reducer and excellent pain reliever.

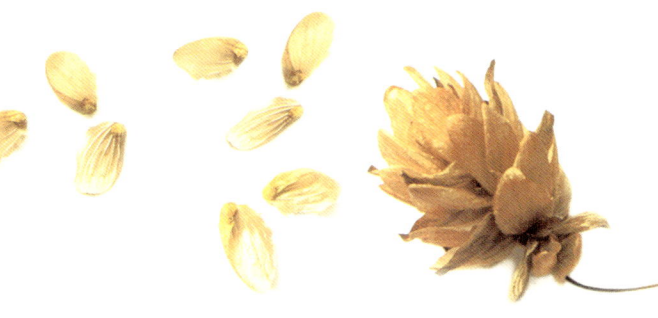

A hop pillow could provide just the solution you need for relief from painful neuralgia.

Olive oil, warmed and dropped into the ear, will provide relief from pain.

GENERAL AILMENTS
Period Pains and PMS

Period pains, also known as dysmenorrhea, are the searing pains felt in the lower abdomen by more than half the female population during a period. About 15% of those women say the pain interferes with their everyday lives. Period pains tend to start during adolescence and become less severe with age—particularly after having a baby.

Cramp-like pains in the lower abdomen at the start of a period are rarely a sign of illness but can cause great misery. Premenstrual syndrome (PMS) affects about 40% of women and causes severe mood swings, headaches, bloating, and sore breasts.

Remedies for Period Pains

Brown rice, wholemeal bread, oats, nuts, and beans will all increase the magnesium, iron,

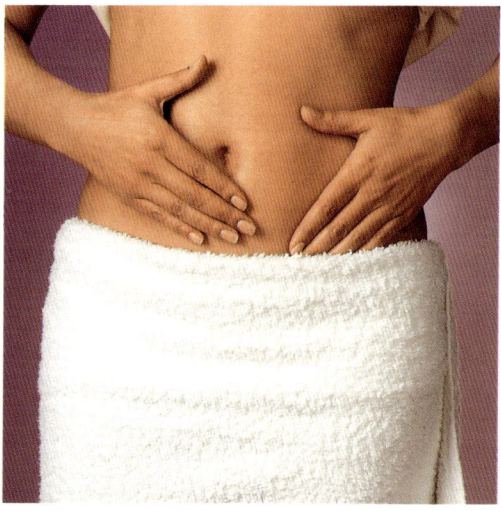

Massage warm castor oil over the lower abdomen to help to ease period pains and relieve the bloating of PMS.

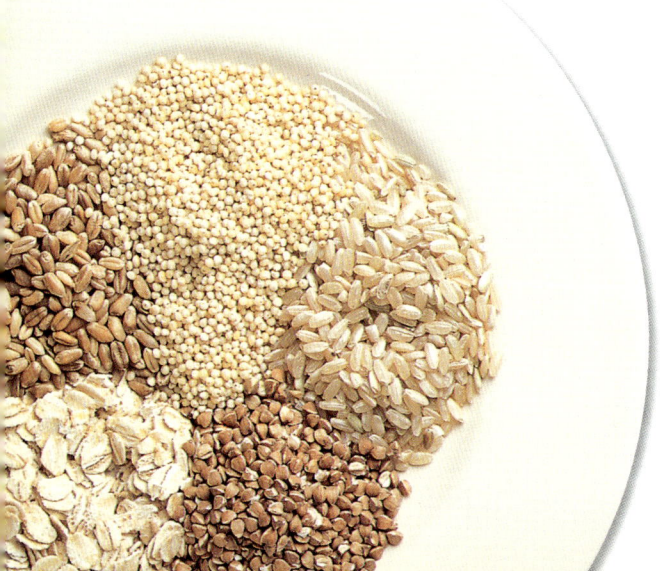

Oats and brown rice help to fight period pains.

zinc, and vitamins in your body, which help you to fight pain. A warm bath with a few drops of chamomile or clary sage essential oils will ease tension and relax muscles. Geranium and rosemary essential oils counter fluid retention.

Angelica is a warming, stimulating herb suitable for women who feel a chill during periods. To make a tea, add one part each of angelica, chamomile, and ginger root to $2\frac{1}{2}$ cups of water and simmer for 15 minutes.

Dandelion is a good source of iron and is one of the best diuretics, supplying plenty of potassium which helps to get rid of excess water. Add young dandelion leaves to a fresh green salad for an appetizing remedy. Yarrow tea can help ease menstrual cramps and decrease menstrual bleeding.

Massage warm castor oil over the lower abdomen. Hot, fresh ginger tea or fresh ginger infused in milk is one of the oldest remedies for period pains. Boil up rhubarb roots into a tea, or try basil tea if you suffer with cramps and particularly heavy periods.

Remedies for PMS

Peppermint tea can help to ease the symptoms of PMS. Freshly cooked asparagus helps to control breast tenderness and bloating. Seaweed may also help—it's the natural iodine that relieves symptoms. Choose wakame, nori, and kombu, and use them in stews or soups.

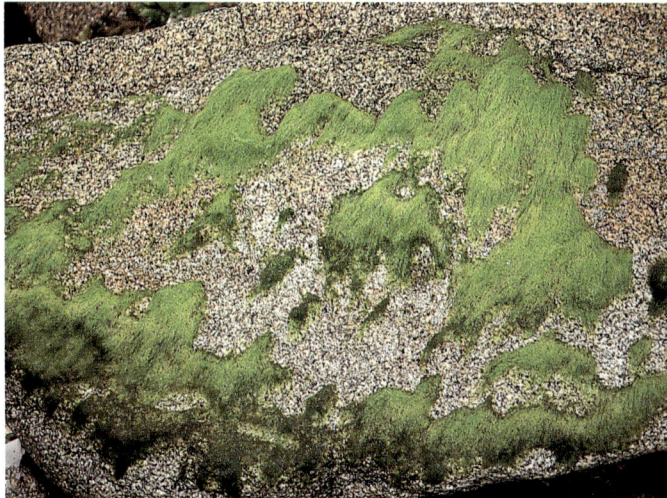

Seaweed contains natural iodine that is useful in relieving PMS symptoms. Edible seaweed is available for use in stews and soups.

A castor oil poultice placed on the lower abdomen will encourage the clearing of toxins through the lymphatic system. Soak an old hand towel in castor oil and place it over the abdomen, cover it with another towel, and place a hot water bottle on top.

Dandelion tea can help with bloating in the run-up to a period. It rids the body of excess fluids. Sage tea also helps, or you can eat either in a leaf salad. Make up a cocktail of spinach, watercress, young nettle shoots, carrots, and beets. Use the raw ingredients in a juicer if you have one, or cook the carrots and beets and process everything in a blender. This combination acts as a wonderful tonic at this time of the month.

Freshly cooked asparagus helps to alleviate the symptoms of breast tenderness and bloating associated with PMS.

GENERAL AILMENTS
Hot Flushes and Menopausal Problems

Hot flushes, night sweats, and mood swings are all symptoms of the menopause, which, although not an illness, can cause untold misery to many women as they get older. Cutting out caffeine is particularly useful for most symptoms of menopause, and there is a range of teas and tisanes which can actively help to relieve symptoms.

Remedies for Hot Flushes

Mint is a famous cooler, so add fresh mint whenever you can to salads. Drink peppermint tea or add some peppermint essential oil to your bathwater.

Sage leaves can be made into a tonic wine that helps to relieve hot flushes.

Sage is known to be the herb of old age. Make up a sage tonic wine by taking a handful of fresh sage leaves and letting them stand in a bottle of good quality white wine for at least two weeks. Sweeten with honey and leave for another week. Strain the liquid through a cloth and bottle it. Drinking a glass before lunch and dinner is most beneficial.

Another great menopause tonic contains borage leaf, lemon balm, raspberry leaf, burdock root, and plantain leaf. All you need to do is to steep the herbs in hot water and drink the liquid during the day in order to lift your spirits.

Celery stalk contains estrogen-stimulating substances that will help with menopausal symptoms.

Pumpkin seeds contain phytoestrogens, which can help with menopausal symptoms.

Remedies for Night Sweats

Drink two cupfuls of sage tea each day. Place three teaspoons of sage leaves in a pan and pour two cups of boiling water over them. Cover and simmer for five minutes. Make it up in the morning and keep it in a thermos for drinking during the day. Ginseng tea is often recommended because it contains plenty of B vitamins and minerals. It also helps boost a flagging libido!

Try marigold tea made from an infusion of flower heads in $4\frac{1}{4}$ cups of boiling water, steeped for ten minutes. Drink it three or four times a day.

Place the leaves of lemon balm under your pillow at night, or drink a cup of lemon balm tea to soothe and revive you.

Remedies for General Symptoms

Calendula, hops, ginseng, sage, and wild yam all have estrogenic action which can be helpful—take these as an infusion or supplement. Eat plenty of rhubarb, oats, and celery stalks which contain similar estrogen-stimulating substances.

Some foods have high levels of phytoestrogens (natural plant estrogens), and these may have a beneficial effect on menopausal symptoms.

Many of these compounds, which are called isoflavones and lignans, are found in soy foods, flax seeds and some herbs.

In Asia, where women eat a diet high in soy foods, they report fewer menopausal symptoms and also have a lower incidence of breast cancer. Some trials have also shown that a diet high in soy decreases the incidence of hot flushes.

Other foods that contain phytoestrogens include mung beans, pumpkin seeds, tofu and tempeh, so try to include these foods in your diet.

Eat plenty of nettles, dandelion, and plantain, which can all be added to salads.

As a general tonic, you could run yourself a hot bath and add essential oils of rosemary or lavender, and this will soothe and refresh you.

Lemon balm leaves, placed under your pillow at night, will soothe you and help you to counter night sweats.

GENERAL AILMENTS
Candida/Thrush

Stress, allergies, too much junk food, and alcohol can all conspire to cause an imbalance in the flora of the gut, colon or vagina, causing the itching and soreness known as candida or thrush. Thrush is a fungal parasite, which can be stimulated by the contraceptive pill or by the use of antibiotics. Simple self-help includes avoiding synthetic underwear or tight jeans and avoiding sex while you have the infection. Oral thrush is more common in babies and children than in adults, and it can be caused by too much sugar in the diet.

Remedies for Vaginal Thrush

Thyme, in the form of a tea, can be used as a douche to ease the discomfort of thrush.

Eat a pot of live yogurt every morning or make up a breakfast of raw oats, live yogurt, and orange juice. A weak solution of one teaspoon of hydrogen peroxide in a glass of warm water, dabbed gently onto the affected area with a swab of cotton wool, will ease the itching.

Live yogurt contains friendly bacteria known as acidophilus, which combat vaginal yeast and other infections caused by this fungus. Put some on a tampon and insert into the vagina (remove within two hours).

Drink honey in cider vinegar each morning, and if you are on a course of antibiotics eat as much raw garlic as you can take for up to a week—it counters most bacterial, fungal, and viral infections. You can even place a peeled clove of garlic wrapped in a little gauze inside the vagina for a powerful local antiseptic effect—it stings like mad, so this one is not for the faint-hearted!

Live yogurt contains friendly bacteria which combat vaginal yeast.

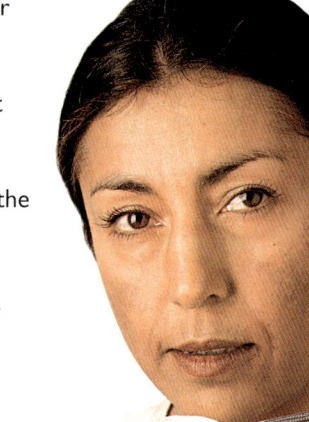

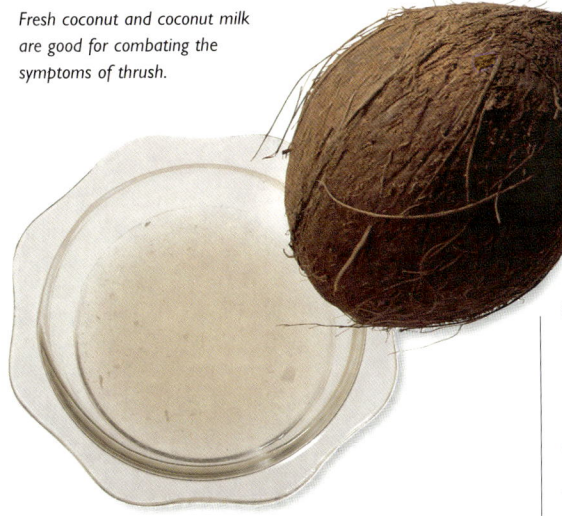

Fresh coconut and coconut milk are good for combating the symptoms of thrush.

solution. Leave the tampon in for four to five hours once or twice a week.

Nasturtium is an age-old remedy for thrush because the flowers act as a natural antibiotic. You could make an infusion from the flowers and use it in a cool bath.

You could make up a douche from $2\frac{1}{2}$ cups of boiled, cooled water to which you have added two drops of lavender oil, or make a douche from chamomile or thyme tea. You can also use either of these mixtures in a shallow bath to ease the discomfort.

Use myrrh or tea tree oil diluted with a teaspoon of vodka and soak a tampon in the

Remedies for Oral Thrush

The best remedies for oral thrush include eating plenty of garlic and lots of live yogurt. Rinse the mouth thoroughly with a solution of apple cider vinegar and warm water with a dash of salt.

Some other foods, such as onions, coconut, and coconut milk, are also thought to be particularly helpful against thrush.

The flowers of the nasturtium act as a natural antibiotic. Use them in an infusion or in a cool bath.

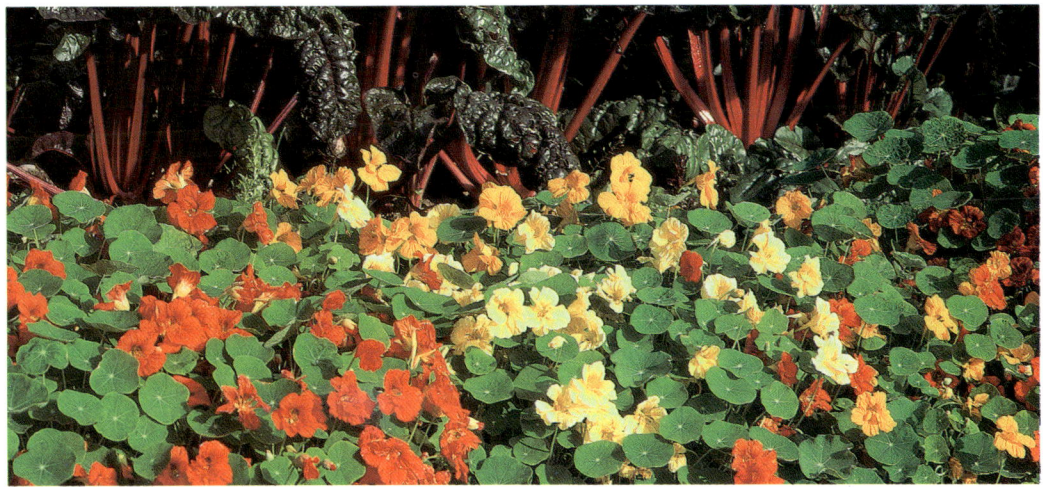

Chilblains, Cramp, and Poor Circulation

Chilblains are a mild form of frostbite and are painful, itchy swellings that generally occur on the hands, feet or ears in response to cold weather. They are usually the result of poor circulation, which can in turn be aggravated by smoking. Some naturopaths believe that cramps and poor circulation are also caused by low potassium or calcium levels.

Remedies for Chilblains

Whatever you do, resist the urge to put your feet on a radiator or a hot water bottle. Get the circulation going by rubbing the feet briskly with a towel.

As long as the skin is not cut or cracked, dust cayenne powder on the chilblains to stimulate blood circulation. If the skin is broken, rub in calendula ointment to promote healing.

One method is to chop up 1lb of turnips in their skins. Boil in 12 cups of water till soft. Soak the affected part in the water while it is still hot but bearable, rubbing pieces of turnip over the inflamed surfaces. The salts and essential oils present in the turnip act as an astringent while also improving the circulation.

Celery stalk contains compounds that lower blood pressure and help to improve circulation.

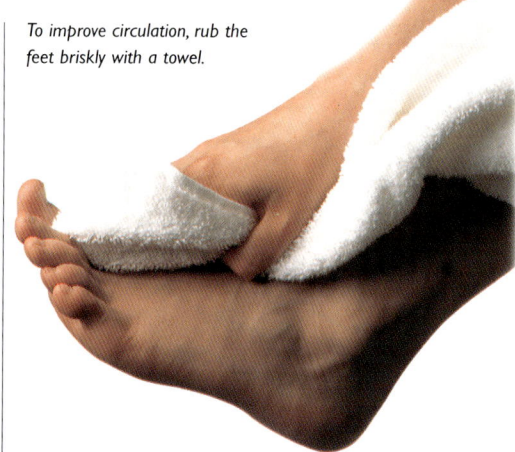

To improve circulation, rub the feet briskly with a towel.

Try fresh horseradish root, bandaged into place. Lemon, garlic or onion juice rubbed on the chilblains can be very effective, or bandage a piece of pithy lemon zest, garlic or onion in place overnight.

Celery stalk is also a good remedy for chilblains. Simmer a bunch of stalks in $4\frac{1}{4}$ cups of water for an hour and soak your feet in a bowl of the mixture for an hour. Make it as hot as you can stand it and try it first thing in the morning and before going to bed.

Remedies for Cramp

Celery stalk contains compounds that reduce high blood pressure by relaxing the smooth muscle lining the blood vessels. The blood flows more freely and pressure drops; this helps cramp symptoms.

Mix one tablespoon of apple cider vinegar and one teaspoon of honey in a glass of warm water. Gulp it down quickly and the discomfort will disappear after only a few minutes.

Much potassium may be lost in many of the commercial brands of vinegar now available, so look out for the unprocessed variety in a health store.

Almonds in the diet will help to reduce the incidence of cramp.

Drink teas that are rich in calcium such as dandelion, raspberry, and plantain leaf. Eat plenty of almonds, sesame seeds, yogurt, and most green vegetables.

"Restless legs" is cramp that causes pain and twitching in the legs. Add seed oils, avocados, and wheatgerm to the diet to alleviate these symptoms. Reduce your meat, high-fat dairy produce and salt intake.

Soak your feet in a solution made from boiled celery stalks to ease chilblains.

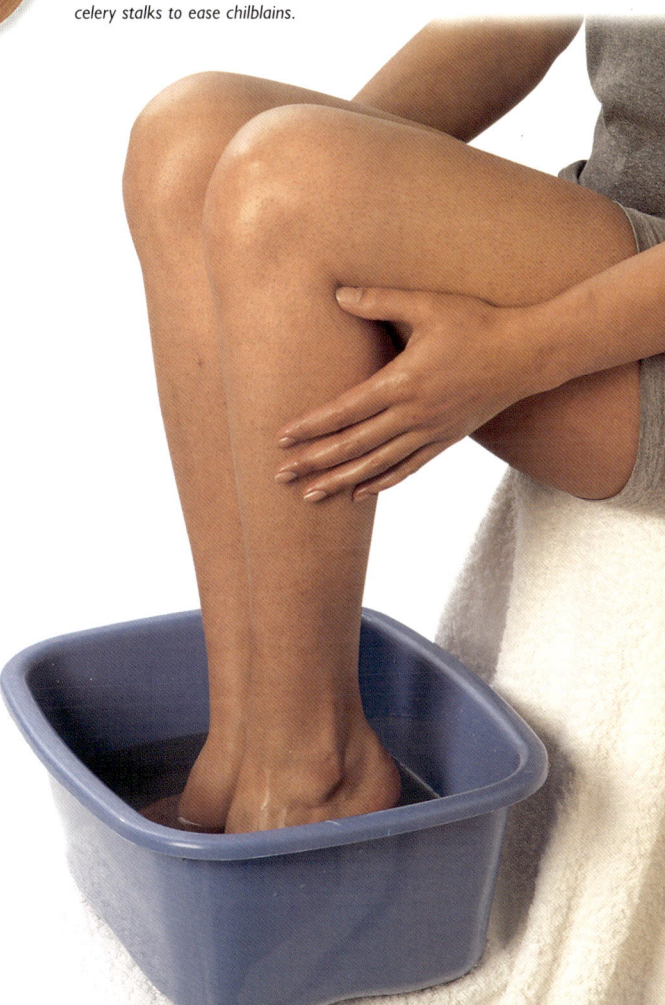

How to Make a Calcium Supplement

- Fill a jar halfway with crushed eggshells.
- Cover with vinegar and allow to sit for two weeks.
- Strain, then take one to three tablespoons daily.
- You can use it as salad dressing or in sauces.
- Sweetened with honey, it can be taken as a refreshing drink.

GENERAL AILMENTS
Eye Conditions

The eye is an incredibly delicate organ and yet it has been built to withstand a large amount of punishment. The anterior part of the eyeball is encased in a tough membrane called the cornea, which can survive and recover from even quite severe injuries. However, alcohol, smoky atmospheres, and working too long at computer screens all conspire to harm, often resulting in sore, itchy or inflamed eyes.

Remedies for Tired Eyes

Rose petals can soothe inflamed or irritated eyelids.

Rose petals are a traditional remedy for inflamed or irritated eyelids. Make up a cooling and soothing compress from two or three petals steeped in a glassful of boiling water for ten minutes. Soak some cotton wool or eyepads in the cooled and strained liquid and place over the eyelids.

Chamomile or marigold tea, used cold as a compress, can also be very healing. Witch hazel, ice-cold from the refrigerator, is very refreshing when your eyes feel tired or you have been staring at a computer all day. Eat plenty of fennel, another marvelous food for tired eyes, or drink it as a tea.

Try an eyebath of three teaspoons of honey diluted in two cups of boiling water and left to cool. Or try a poultice of cabbage leaves, softened but not cooked in boiling water. You may look ridiculous with the leaves over your eyelids but it really works. A raw potato or cucumber placed over closed eyelids can have the same effect.

Borage was valued by the ancient Greeks for strengthening weak eyes and preventing cataracts. You are more likely to develop cataracts if your diet is lacking in beta-carotene, folic acid, and vitamin C. Borage contains all three, so it is a good idea to try to incorporate it in your diet.

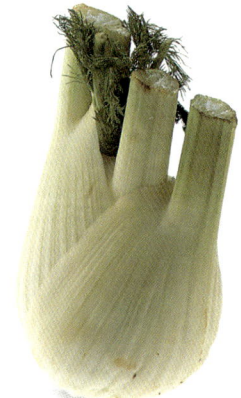

Include plenty of fennel in your diet; it is marvelous for tired eyes.

Remedies for Styes

An eyebath of warm boracic lotion or a poultice of fresh, steamed cabbage leaves will disperse a stye. Or try a drop each of the essential oils of lavender and lemon with a teaspoon of cooled boiled water and bathe the eye with the solution. This will also ease the symptoms of conjunctivitis.

Second World War pilots were encouraged to eat plenty of carrots to improve their night vision.

Past Beliefs

Carrots were once believed to be a super-food for eyes, and pilots during the Second World War were officially encouraged to eat plenty. In the old days, anything golden was reputed to benefit the sight, including gazing at marigolds during the day.

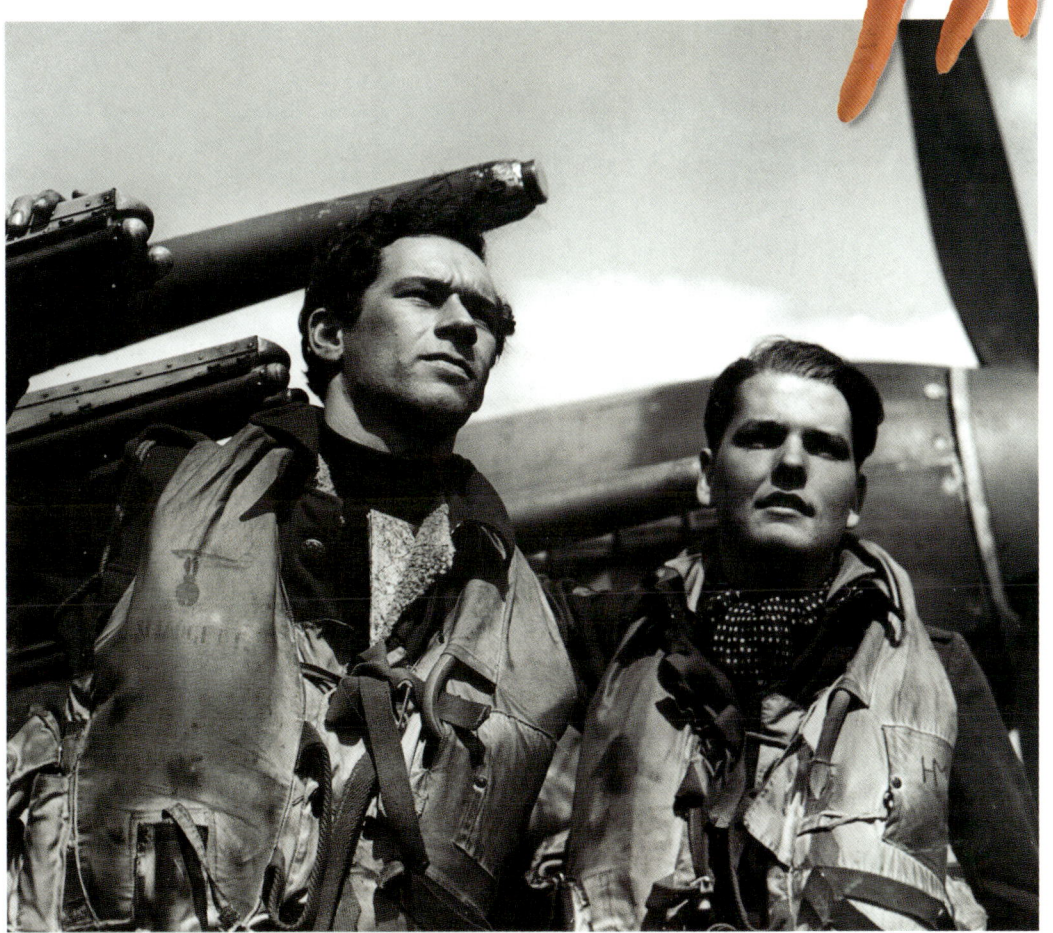

GENERAL AILMENTS
Insomnia

In these stressful times it is hardly any wonder that many people find it hard to get to sleep at night. However, there are certain things you can do to promote a good night's sleep. Try to relax before going to bed, and avoid coffee and alcohol, which tend to keep you awake rather than promote good sleep. Take a warm bath with Epsom salts or play some quiet music. Have a bedtime ritual, so your brain learns to slow down before you settle down to sleep.

Remedies for Insomnia

Natives of certain parts of Italy reputedly slept with cloves of garlic between their toes to ensure a good night's sleep! The Victorians, on the other hand, favored washing the head with dill or placing dill on the pillow at night.

Adding two teaspoons of apple cider vinegar and two teaspoons of honey to a glass of hot water and drinking it at bedtime may seem a little more user-friendly. Try placing a few drops of lavender oil on the pulse points of the wrist and forehead before you go to bed—it

Eating plenty of lettuce will help you get a good night's sleep.

has a soothing and calming effect. Place celery seeds in a piece of cheesecloth and inhale the fumes as you settle down for the night.

Lettuce is supposed to contain sleep-inducing compounds, so eat it raw or drink a lettuce infusion. Mandarin oranges also have

To help combat insomnia, place some drops of lavender oil on the wrists and forehead before settling down for the night.

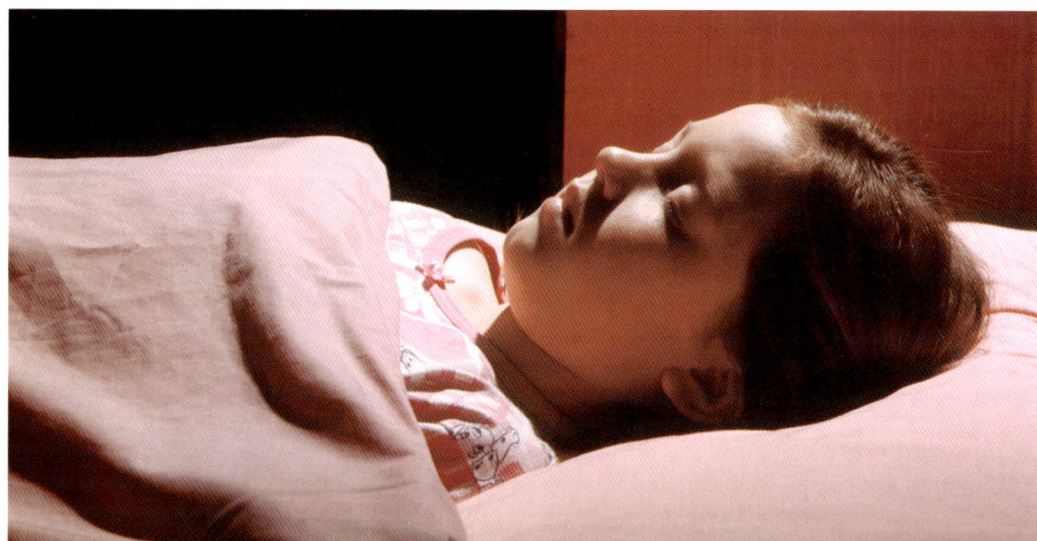

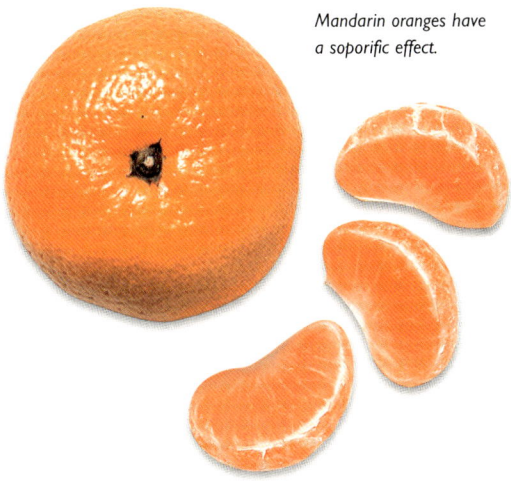

Mandarin oranges have a soporific effect.

Make up your own version with the juice of two oranges in a little hot water sweetened with honey.

A footbath is a good way to bring on sleep because it encourages the blood to flow from the head to the feet. Mix up some lavender and rosemary essential oils and add to a bowl of warm water. A mustard footbath can work just as well.

Warm milk and honey sprinkled with a pinch of cinnamon helps prepare children for sleep.

a soporific effect—it is a good idea to eat one after your evening meal.

You could make up a tea from elderberry flowers, which are thought to relax the nerves and induce sleep.

Native Americans used to eat raw onions to get a good night's sleep. They also made a sleep potion from poppy heads infused in hot water. If this seems a little drastic, try valerian tea just before going to bed.

Make up this infusion: put the ground seeds from one cardamom pod, two drops of peppermint oil, one teaspoon of sugar and a pinch of baking soda in a cup of boiling water and drink while it is still hot.

Add a teaspoon of honey to a cup of warm milk and sprinkle with cinnamon: this is a good drink for helping wakeful children go to sleep.

Orange flower water was a traditional cure for insomnia among English gentlewomen.

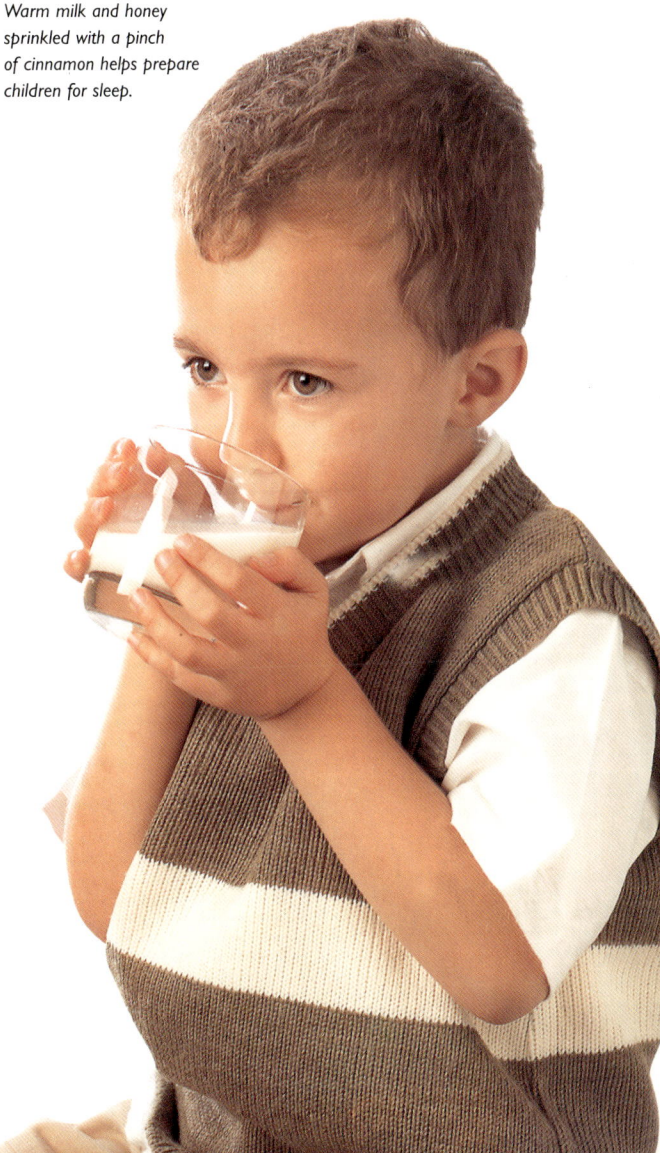

Foot and Hand Care

We have no respect for our feet—we cram them into badly fitting shoes, encase them in synthetic fabrics and demand they perform their task tirelessly, supporting us for hours on end. No wonder we suffer from all sorts of foot complaints, from bunions, calluses, and corns to unpleasant fungal infections such as athlete's foot. Although we are kinder to our hands, we still think nothing of dipping them in and out of hot water all day, which can result in chapped skin or dry nails.

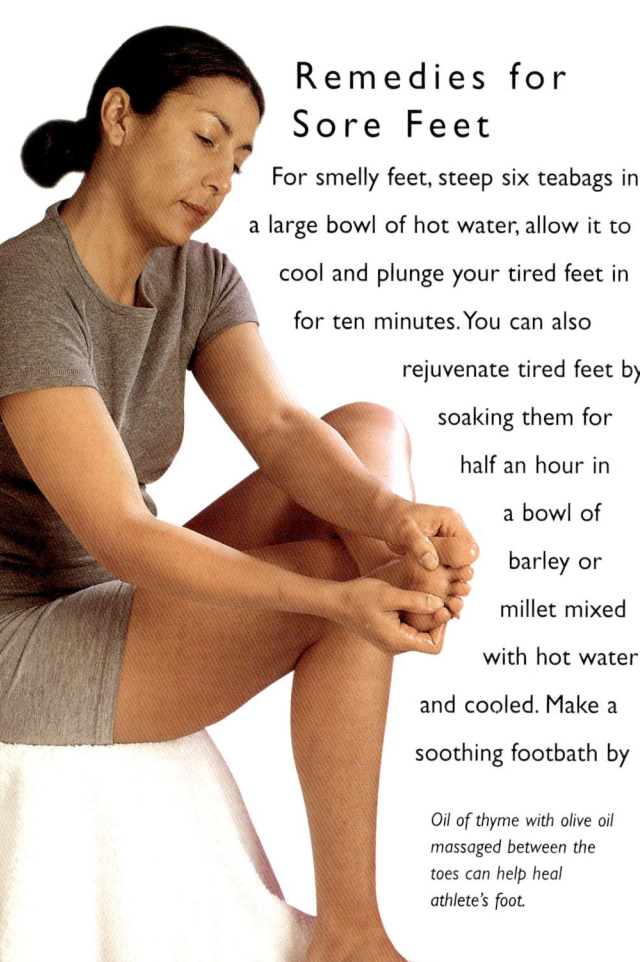

Remedies for Sore Feet

For smelly feet, steep six teabags in a large bowl of hot water, allow it to cool and plunge your tired feet in for ten minutes. You can also rejuvenate tired feet by soaking them for half an hour in a bowl of barley or millet mixed with hot water and cooled. Make a soothing footbath by

Oil of thyme with olive oil massaged between the toes can help heal athlete's foot.

We need to have more respect for our poor old feet! Give them a soothing footbath or massage them with essential oils as a treat.

adding one tablespoon of sea salt to a basin of warm water. In cold weather add a teaspoon of mustard powder to warm them up.

Remedies for Corns

Rub corns with castor oil daily for two weeks to get rid of them completely. Put a piece of lemon zest or raw tomato over the corn and cover with a bandage. The juice of the fruit will soften the corn overnight. The same can be done by soaking leeks in water or vinegar for 24 hours and then applying as a poultice. Make a soothing footbath by adding four or five drops of peppermint oil to a bowl of tepid water. You can also use a couple of peppermint teabags infused for ten minutes.

Remedies for Athlete's Foot

Make up a mixture of equal parts vinegar and warm water or surgical spirit and bathe the feet in a bowl. Massage between the toes with natural yogurt, leaving it to soak in overnight. Add a few drops of essential oil of thyme or rosemary to some olive oil and massage the feet carefully between the toes.

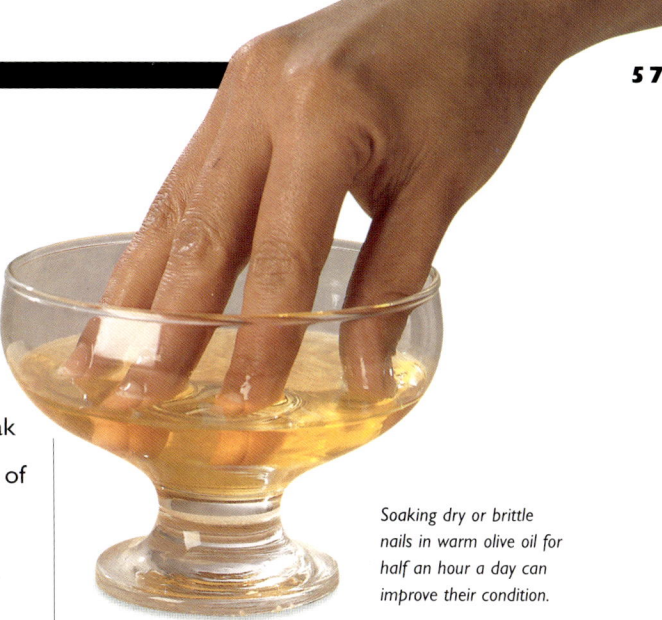

Soaking dry or brittle nails in warm olive oil for half an hour a day can improve their condition.

Remedies for Verrucas and Warts

Peel the skin of a potato as thinly as possible. Rub the inner side of the skin on the wart twice a day. Thanks to a chemical in the potato near the skin, the wart should turn black and drop off within a couple of weeks.

The milky juice squeezed from the stem of a dandelion or celandine can also be used as a balm. Smooth it onto the affected area and cover with a plaster. The next morning the wart or verruca should have disappeared.

Remedy for Dry Hands

Mix together $\frac{1}{4}$ cup of ground almonds, a beaten egg, a handful of comfrey root and a tablespoon of honey. Coat your hands with the mixture and pull on an old pair of leather or cotton gloves and wear overnight. Rinse hands in the morning and repeat this for a week. Your hands will feel very soft and supple.

Remedies for Brittle and Stained Nails

Immerse dry or brittle nails in warm olive oil for 30 minutes a day until you see an improvement.

To remove stains, rub the hands and nails with the pithy side of a piece of lemon zest, leave for a minute and then wash off.

A mixture of ground almonds, egg, comfrey, and honey may be just the moisturizer your hands need.

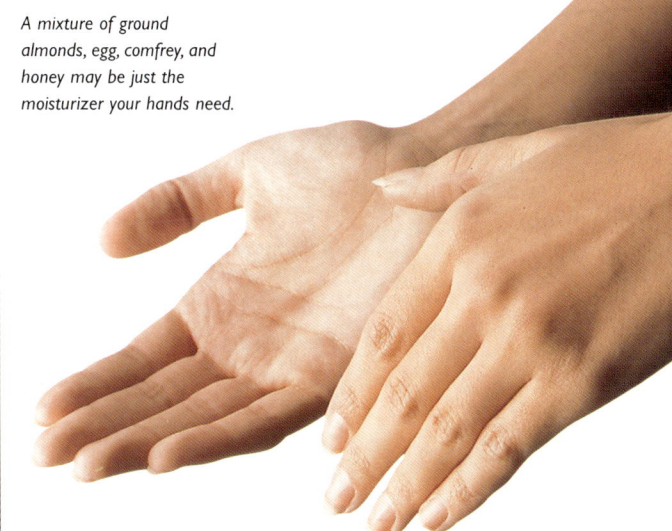

Shampoos, "Feel Good" Treatments, and Tonics

We tend to forget that many natural beauty treatments have been used through the ages for all sorts of cleansing creams and lotions. Cleopatra was reputed to have used aloe vera as a moisturizer, and today most proprietary brands of moisturizing cream contain this substance. Almond oil is another great skin softener—you can add whatever essential oil you feel appropriate to smoothe and pamper your skin. The condition of your hair and scalp can be affected by your general state of health, so almost any stressful condition will cause your skin and hair to appear lifeless and dull. A balanced diet is the basis of good health, hair, and skin, but here are some extra tips to give nature a helping hand!

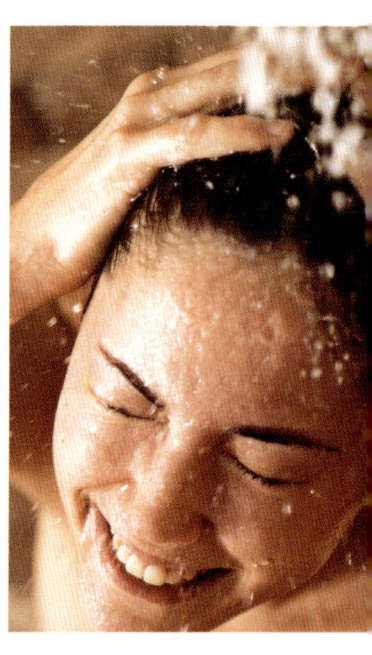

Pamper yourself with a natural, homemade shampoo or "feel good" treatment and improve your general sense of wellbeing.

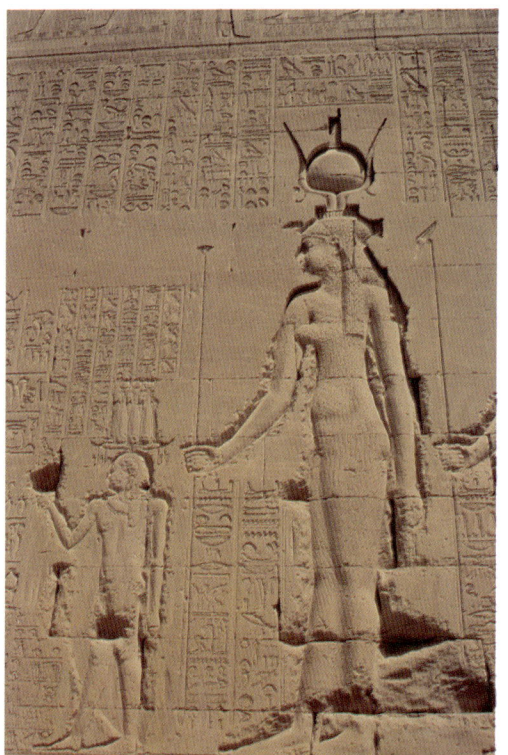

Remedies for Dry Hair

To keep your hair in top condition, try massaging a few drops of oil of rosemary into the scalp then rinsing with an infusion of nettles. For very dry hair, warm two tablespoons of olive oil in a cup placed in a pan of hot water. Massage the oil into the scalp. Steep a towel in hot water, wring it out and wrap it around your head for about two

Even the ancient Egyptians needed a little help to stay beautiful! Cleopatra was reputed to have used aloe vera as a moisturizer.

hours. Rinse with a solution of half a cupful of cider vinegar to 11 cups of water.

Make an egg shampoo for dry hair. Use 1 tablespoon of fresh rosemary, $2\frac{1}{2}$ cups of hot water and one egg. Steep the rosemary in the water for 20 minutes and allow to cool. Beat in the egg. Massage into the hair and rinse well.

Remedies for Dandruff

Cut a lemon in half and rub the two halves into the scalp. Leave for ten minutes, then wash the hair. Sour milk has the same effect but will not smell as nice.

Wrap one or two pieces of fresh ginger root in cheesecloth. Boil it up in $2\frac{1}{2}$ cups of water. After shampooing, rinse your hair with the liquid, massaging it into the hair.

Rinse your hair with cider vinegar, wrap your head in a towel and leave for half an hour. Rinse out completely. Repeat three times a week until the dandruff disappears.

Remedy for Split Ends

Comb in a mixture of equal quantities of warmed castor oil and olive oil. Follow this by shampooing with an egg yolk. Wrap your head up in a warm towel and let the egg yolk soak in for at least an hour.

Aloe vera has been used in moisturizers through the ages and is still used today.

Then add half a cup of cider vinegar to 20 cups of cool water and rinse the mixture through your hair, followed by a cool rinse with clear water to remove all traces. For thinning hair, rinse your hair with flat beer.

"Feel Good" Tonics

Make yourself a natural tonic. Some people swear by drinking a teaspoon of apple cider vinegar and a teaspoon of honey in $\frac{3}{4}$–1 cups of hot water mid-morning and mid-afternoon. It provides a boost of energy which carries them through to the next meal.

Or try making up a purifying tonic by mixing a tablespoon of crushed blueberries and a tablespoon of shredded watercress with $1\frac{1}{4}$ cups of boiling water poured over. Cover the liquid and leave to cool, then strain it. Drink a cup twice a day. It's guaranteed to make you feel a million dollars.

You can make an egg shampoo with rosemary—it works wonders for dry hair problems.

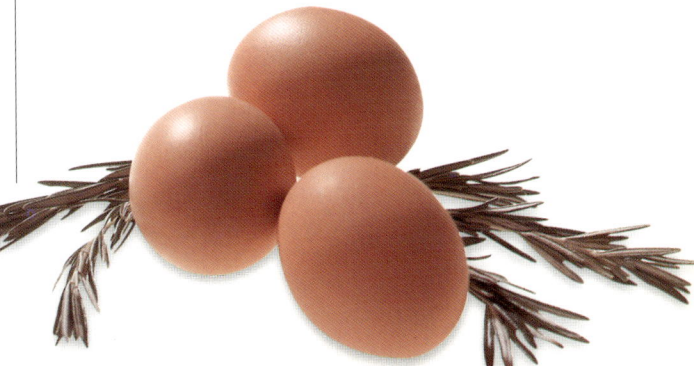

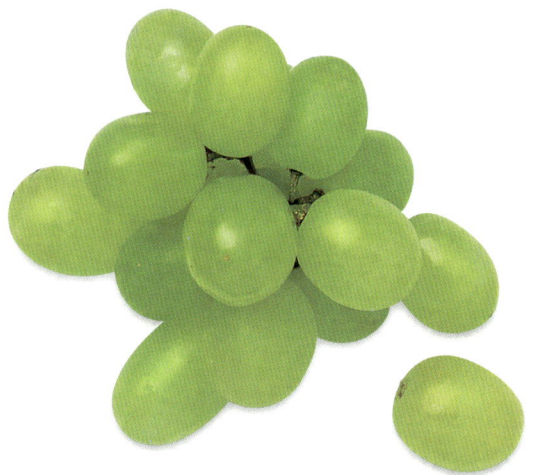

Green grapes can be used in a homemade facial cleanser.

For a dandelion tonic, pick enough dandelion flower heads to make 5 cups of petals. Cut off the stem and collar at the end of each flower. Rinse the dandelions in water before preparing the petals. Place the petals in a pan, cover with 11 cups of water and boil for 20 minutes. Add two oranges and two lemons. Add a spoonful of baker's yeast and allow to stand for 48 hours before straining through cheesecloth. Add 3lb of sugar and stir well. Use as a feel good tonic whenever you need one.

For the Face

You can make a natural cleansing cream with eight tablespoons of beeswax heated up with 2 cups of liquid paraffin. Add $1\frac{1}{4}$ cups of water to the wax and oil mixture, stirring continuously. Leave it to cool and transfer it to jars for storage.

To make a cleanser, mix ten green grapes, two teaspoons of apple cider vinegar, one teaspoon of honey and a teaspoon of oatmeal in a blender until the liquid becomes sticky. Clean your face and neck in your usual way and apply the mixture, leaving it on for at least five minutes. Rinse with warm water and pat dry.

Lemons are marvelous for greasy skin that is prone to blackheads—you can drink the juice and also apply it to the skin. Its high antioxidant content makes it an excellent treatment for wrinkles too. Dilute it with mineral water and massage it gently at the first sign of wrinkles, particularly around the mouth and eyes.

To make a face pack for greasy skin, pit and mash a large cucumber, add a teaspoon of lemon juice, a teaspoon of witch hazel, an egg white and two tablespoons of cream or plain yogurt and blend all the ingredients in a blender. Apply the mixture to the face and leave for 20 to 30 minutes until nearly dry, then rinse well with warm water.

For a great face mask, mix an equal

Make up a face pack for greasy skin from natural ingredients such as cucumber.

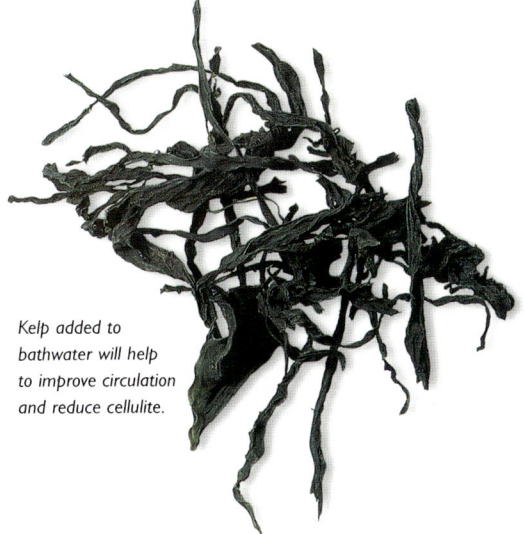

Kelp added to bathwater will help to improve circulation and reduce cellulite.

quantity of oatmeal and ground almonds into a paste by adding enough liquid to thicken the mixture and smooth onto the face and neck. Add one teaspoon of wheatgerm or brewer's yeast for dry skin, or kaolin to draw out spots and impurities.

If you have problem skin, Fuller's earth (a clay available at drug stores) will help an oily skin and stimulate the blood supply. Witch hazel, beaten egg white, yogurt or lemon juice will all help to dry up an oily skin. Egg yolk, honey, soured cream, pulped bananas or avocado will all benefit a dry skin. Rosemary oil added to a base of oats and almonds will invigorate a tired, dull-looking skin.

You could use the pulp of the pawpaw fruit to rub over the face and this will help to slough off dead skin cells.

A tablespoon of castor oil mixed with two tablespoons of almond oil makes an excellent eye make-up remover.

For Cellulite

Cellulite is the term used to describe the puckered areas of fatty flesh, often referred to as "orange peel skin," that generally occur around the tops of the thighs, hips, buttocks, and upper arms, and is more common in women than men. No one really knows what causes cellulite, yet theories abound on how it can be treated.

Fresh parsley is a rich source of vitamin C, a good detoxifier, and a diuretic, so it helps the body eliminate excess water. Eat plenty of the raw herb in salads.

Boil up the zest of a lemon in water and leave it overnight. You then drink it first thing in the morning.

Use kelp in your bathwater—it boosts the circulation. Dandelion tea will rid the body of any excess fluid.

Chop two handfuls of ivy leaves and mix with four handfuls of bran and enough warm water to make a paste. This can then be applied to the affected areas as a poultice.

The pulp of the pawpaw fruit will slough off dead skin cells.

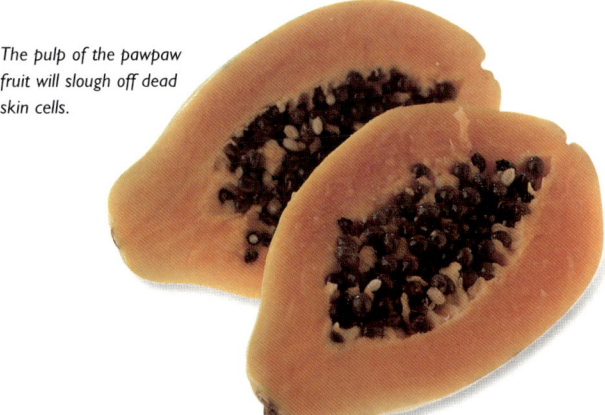

Useful Home Remedies

Almond oil: as a base for massage and rubs; for earache

Aloe vera: as a facial cleanser

Angelica: use the leaves or roots as a diuretic, expectorant, antispasmodic; digestive tonic for children's coughs and colds; for fainting fits; for a fever

Asparagus: for eczema

Avocado: as a hand cream; as a cleanser; for sunburn; for cuts and grazes; for acne

Baking soda: for sunburn; for cystitis

Bananas: for diarrhea

Barley: for cystitis

Basil: as an antiseptic

Beet: for fever; to clear the blood; for acne

Blackberry leaves: for diarrhea; for food poisoning

Blackcurrants: for infection and inflammation

Blueberries: for cystitis; for diarrhea; for mouth ulcers and sore gums

Borage: for coughs; for constipation; as a diuretic

Buttermilk: for sunburn

Cabbage: for arthritis and rheumatism; as a poultice for back pain; as a detoxifier; for asthma; for constipation

Camphor oil: stimulant or sedative; antiseptic, can be used on cuts and grazes; for lumbago

Carrots: for stomach disorders; for cleansing the system; for eye problems; for asthma; for constipation

Castor oil: for food poisoning

Cayenne pepper: as a poultice for joint irritation; with garlic for a bad sore throat

Celandine: for jaundice, throat infections, verrucas and warts, failing eyesight

Celery: for urinary tract infections

Chili peppers: for rheumatism

Cider vinegar: can be used for practically anything. It cures fungal infections, stomach infections and can be used in a footbath for athlete's foot

Cinnamon: a warming digestive, antispasmodic and antiseptic; good for menstrual cramps and for diarrhea; with ginger for a chesty cough

Cloves: as a painkiller for toothache and to ease wasp stings; can also help nausea; for a fever

Comfrey: for bruises and sprains

Cowslip: contains salicin (like aspirin)

Cranberries: the perfect answer to cystitis

Cream: for wounds

Cucumber: with glycerine for burns; for headaches

Dandelion: a diuretic and can be used to cleanse the whole system of toxins; good for mosquito bites

Dock leaves: for nettle stings

Echinacea: an antibiotic; for colds and flu

Egg yolk: for a gravel graze; for a hangover; for lumbago

Elderberries: for burns and sunburn; for coughs; for earache; for fever; for headaches; for insomnia; for toothaches; for neuralgia

Epsom salts: for back pain; for infections; for menstrual pain

Fennel: for bad breath; for indigestion; for constipation; for colds and flu; as a diuretic

Feverfew: for migraine

Figs: for constipation

Friar's balsam: as an inhalant for allergies, eg, asthma and hay fever; for cuts and grazes

Fuller's earth: clay for use as a face pack to draw impurities from the skin

Garlic: as a natural antibiotic and antiseptic; for cleaning wounds; for stomach disorders; for cleansing the blood; for corns; for coughs; for earache; for diarrhea; for hangovers; for thrush; for verrucas; as an insect repellent

Ginger: for arthritis and rheumatism; for colds and circulation problems; in a footbath for headaches and migraine

Grapefruit: for psoriasis

Hibiscus: for a fever

Honey: for asthma and allergies; for constipation; for coughs, colds and fever; for sore throats; for cuts and grazes

Honeycomb: chewed for allergies

Hops: for insomnia; for headaches

Horseradish: for acne; for chilblains; for mosquito bites; for sinuses

Hyssop: in tea to support the immune system

Irish moss: for asthma

Ivy: for cellulite; for sciatica

Lavender: for acne; for burns; for coughs and colds; for earache; for a hangover; in a hair treatment; for menstrual cramps; for rheumatism; for the skin; for thrush; for sprains

Lemon: for colds; as a digestive; for fever; in hair and skin treatments; for teeth; for stings

Lemon balm: for burns

Lemon juice: for sunburn; for bites and stings

Linseed: in a poultice for bursitis

Marigold: for bruises and burns; for sore gums

Marshmallow: for bursitis; for eczema

Milk: in rice pudding for diarrhea; with cinnamon for insomnia
Milk of magnesia: for indigestion; for sunburn

Mud and clay: for sunburn

Mustard: as a rub for bad backs; in a footbath for colds or flu

Nettles: as a diuretic; for cleansing the blood; for eliminating toxins; in soup for insomnia

Oats: for stress; for cleansing the blood; in a poultice for cellulite; for menopause and period pains

Olive oil: for food poisoning

Onions: for colds; for cystitis; to help digestion; for allergies

Oregano: for migraine

Parsley: for bad breath; as a diuretic

Pepper: for toothache

Peppermint: for nausea; for colds and fever; for headache; for menopause; as a mosquito repellent; for IBS

Plums: for psoriasis

Potato: for stomach disorders; for sore eyes; as an anti-inflammatory; for IBS

Prunes: for constipation; for psoriasis

Rice: for bowel disorders, especially diarrhea

Rosemary: as a disinfectant; for fever; for headaches; in hair treatments; as a mouthwash; for rheumatism

Rose petals: as an eye treatment

Sage: for thrush; for menopause; for mouth/gums; for sore throats

Salt: as a gargle for sore throats; for fungal infections; in water for cuts and grazes

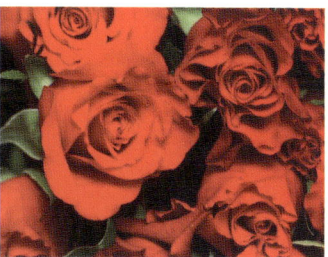

Sandalwood: in a bath for a hangover

Slippery elm: for indigestion; for bursitis

Soya: for menopausal symptoms

Strawberries: as a laxative for constipation

Thyme: for colds; as a disinfectant in a footbath; as an infusion for improving a hoarse voice

Tomatoes (canned): for migraine

Turmeric: for sprains; for rheumatism

Turnips: for coughs and colds; (boiled) for cystitis

Umeboshi plums: for food poisoning; for hangovers

Watercress: for acne

Willow: for toothache

Wine: for hangovers; garlic wine as a tonic

Witch hazel: first-line treatment for cuts and grazes; as a deodorant; for hemorrhoids

Yogurt: for cuts and grazes; for thrush

Index